GLYCEMIC GOODNESS

Wholesome Recipes for Balanced Living

MITT Creations

Copyright © 2023 MITT Creations.

Table of Content

Please note that the recipes and information provided in this book are intended for general informational purposes only and are not a substitute for professional medical advice. Always consult with a qualified healthcare provider or registered dietitian before making significant changes to your diet, especially if you have specific health conditions or dietary needs.

Introduction

Welcome to the "Glycemic Index Diet Cookbook" - your comprehensive guide to exploring the world of delicious and nutritious meals that align with the principles of the Glycemic Index (GI) diet. Whether you're seeking to manage blood sugar levels, improve overall health, or simply enjoy flavorful dishes, this cookbook is your ticket to a culinary journey that focuses on smart carbohydrate choices and balanced nutrition.

The Glycemic Index is a powerful tool that ranks carbohydrates based on their impact on blood sugar levels. By incorporating low-GI foods into your diet, you can achieve stable blood sugar levels, better energy management, and improved overall well-being. With this cookbook, we invite you to embark on a delicious adventure where every recipe is carefully crafted to support your health goals.

In the pages ahead, you'll find an array of mouthwatering recipes that showcase the versatility and diversity of low-GI ingredients. From hearty breakfasts to satisfying dinners and delectable desserts, each dish is thoughtfully designed to bring you maximum flavor and nutritional benefits. You'll discover an abundance of fruits, vegetables, whole grains, lean proteins, and healthy fats that will nourish your body from the inside out.

Whether you're a seasoned cook or a culinary novice, this cookbook provides step-by-step instructions and cooking tips to make your journey in the kitchen a delightful and rewarding experience. Additionally, you'll gain valuable insights into the fundamentals of the Glycemic Index, empowering you to make informed food choices and embrace a healthier lifestyle.

Before you dive into the recipes, we encourage you to take a moment to familiarize yourself with the essential principles of the Glycemic Index and its impact on your health. Let this cookbook be your guide as you embark on a path of flavorful and nourishing meals that will not only tantalize your taste buds but also promote well-being and vitality.

Get ready to savor the flavors, explore the benefits, and embrace the culinary delights of the Glycemic Index Diet Cookbook. Your journey to a healthier, happier you starts here!

Understanding the Glycemic Index

The Glycemic Index (GI) is a valuable tool that measures how different carbohydrate-containing foods affect our blood sugar levels. It ranks carbohydrates on a scale from 0 to 100 based on their ability to raise blood glucose levels. Foods with a high GI (70 or above) cause rapid spikes in blood sugar, leading to a quick energy surge followed by a crash. On the other hand, foods with a low GI (55 or below) cause a gradual and sustained increase in blood sugar, providing steady energy levels.

Comprehending the GI is crucial, especially for individuals with diabetes, as it helps them make informed food choices that support blood sugar management. However, the GI is not just for those with diabetes; it can benefit anyone striving for better overall health and stable energy levels.

Low-GI foods include non-starchy vegetables, legumes, whole grains, and most fruits. These options are rich in fiber, vitamins, and minerals, promoting satiety and providing essential nutrients. High-GI foods, such as refined grains, sugary treats, and some processed snacks, should be consumed in moderation as they can lead to rapid spikes in blood sugar and contribute to insulin resistance.

By incorporating low-GI foods into our diets, we can maintain stable blood sugar levels, curb cravings, and enhance our overall well-being. Understanding the Glycemic Index empowers us to make conscious food choices that promote sustained energy, support weight management, and contribute to a balanced and healthy lifestyle.

What is the Glycemic Index?

The Glycemic Index (GI) is a valuable tool that measures how different carbohydrate-containing foods affect our blood sugar levels. It ranks carbohydrates on a scale from 0 to 100 based on their ability to raise blood glucose levels. Foods with a high GI (70 or above) cause rapid spikes in blood sugar, leading to a quick energy surge followed by a crash. On the other hand, foods with a low GI (55 or below) cause a gradual and sustained increase in blood sugar, providing steady energy levels.

The concept of the Glycemic Index was first developed by Dr. David Jenkins and his team at the University of Toronto in the early 1980s. Their research aimed to better understand how different carbohydrates impacted blood sugar levels, particularly in individuals with diabetes. Since then, the GI has become a widely recognized tool for individuals seeking to manage blood sugar levels, promote weight control, and improve overall health.

Low-GI foods include non-starchy vegetables, legumes, whole grains, and most fruits. These options are rich in fiber, vitamins, and minerals, promoting satiety and providing essential nutrients. High-GI foods, such as refined grains, sugary treats, and some processed snacks, should be consumed in moderation as they can lead to rapid spikes in blood sugar and contribute to insulin resistance.

By incorporating low-GI foods into our diets, we can maintain stable blood sugar levels, curb cravings, and enhance our overall well-being. Understanding the Glycemic Index empowers us to make conscious food choices that promote sustained energy, support weight management, and contribute to a balanced and healthy lifestyle.

How Does the Glycemic Index Work?

The Glycemic Index (GI) is a valuable tool that provides insight into how different carbohydrate-containing foods impact our blood sugar levels. Understanding how the GI works is essential for making informed food choices, especially for individuals with diabetes or those striving for better overall health.

The GI operates on a scale from 0 to 100, with pure glucose serving as the reference point at 100. Foods with a high GI, such as white bread, processed cereals, and sugary snacks, are rapidly digested and absorbed, leading to a sharp increase in blood glucose levels. This rapid spike causes a surge in energy but is often followed by a sudden drop, leaving individuals feeling fatigued and craving more carbohydrates.

On the other hand, foods with a low GI, like most non-starchy vegetables, whole grains, and legumes, are digested and absorbed more slowly. This gradual release of glucose into the bloodstream leads to a more stable and sustained increase in blood sugar levels. As a result, individuals experience a steady flow of energy and are less likely to experience drastic fluctuations in mood and appetite.

Factors that influence a food's GI include its physical structure, the presence of fiber, fat, and protein, as well as food processing and cooking methods. Combining foods with different GI values can also impact the overall GI of a meal, as certain components can slow down the digestion and absorption of carbohydrates.

The GI is a valuable tool for those managing diabetes, as it can help them make choices that support stable blood sugar levels. Additionally, incorporating more low-GI foods into the diet is beneficial for everyone, promoting sustained energy, reducing the risk of chronic diseases, and supporting overall well-being. By understanding how the Glycemic Index works, individuals can make informed dietary decisions that align with their health goals and contribute to a balanced and nourishing lifestyle.

Benefits of the Glycemic Index Diet

The Glycemic Index (GI) diet offers a myriad of benefits for individuals seeking to improve their overall health and well-being. By understanding and incorporating the principles of the GI diet into their eating habits, individuals can experience a range of positive effects that support both physical and mental health.

One of the primary benefits of the GI diet is its impact on blood sugar management. Consuming foods with a low GI helps regulate blood glucose levels, reducing the risk of sudden spikes and crashes. This steady control of blood sugar provides sustained energy, curbs cravings, and helps individuals maintain a more stable mood throughout the day.

Furthermore, the GI diet has shown promise in weight management and weight loss efforts. Low-GI foods generally promote a feeling of fullness and satiety, leading to reduced hunger and a decreased likelihood of overeating. By incorporating more low-GI foods into their meals, individuals may find it easier to control their calorie intake and achieve their weight-related goals.

Additionally, the GI diet has been associated with improved heart health. Consuming fewer high-GI foods, which are often linked to inflammation and insulin resistance, can reduce the risk of developing cardiovascular diseases. Instead, the focus on low-GI options, such as whole grains and fruits, provides essential nutrients and fiber that support heart health.

Another advantage of the GI diet is its potential to enhance cognitive function and mental well-being. Stable blood sugar levels can help maintain focus, concentration, and memory. Moreover, the diet's emphasis on whole, nutrient-dense foods can positively influence brain health and reduce the risk of cognitive decline over time.

In conclusion, the Glycemic Index diet offers numerous benefits for individuals aiming to optimize their health and manage certain health conditions. By incorporating low-GI foods and making conscious dietary choices, individuals can experience improved blood sugar control, support their weight management efforts, enhance heart health, and enjoy the long-term benefits of a balanced and nourishing lifestyle.

Chapter 1

Getting Started with the Glycemic Index Diet

Embarking on the journey of the Glycemic Index (GI) diet can be an empowering step towards better health and well-being. Whether you are seeking to manage blood sugar levels, improve energy levels, or support weight management, the GI diet offers a wealth of benefits. To get started on the right foot, here are some essential steps and guidelines to follow:

Assess Your Current Eating Habits: Begin by evaluating your current diet and identifying high-GI foods that may be contributing to blood sugar spikes and energy fluctuations. Take note of refined carbohydrates, sugary snacks, and processed foods, which often rank high on the GI scale.

Understand the Basics of the Glycemic Index: Familiarize yourself with the GI scale, which ranges from 0 to 100. Foods with a high GI (70 or above) cause rapid increases in blood sugar levels, while low-GI foods (55 or below) result in a more gradual and steady rise.

Create a Balanced Meal Plan: Craft a meal plan that incorporates a variety of low-GI foods, such as non-starchy vegetables, whole grains, legumes, and fruits. Pair these foods with lean proteins and healthy fats to create balanced and satisfying meals.

Choose Smart Carbohydrate Choices: Opt for carbohydrates that have a lower impact on blood sugar, such as sweet potatoes, quinoa, and berries. These choices provide essential nutrients and promote longer-lasting energy.

Learn to Read Food Labels: Familiarize yourself with food labels and look for products with lower glycemic loads. Focus on whole foods and minimize consumption of highly processed items.

Be Mindful of Food Combinations: Combining high-GI and low-GI foods in a meal can affect the overall GI of the meal. Pair high-GI foods with fiber-rich options to slow down digestion and reduce the overall glycemic impact.

Embrace Whole Foods: Make whole, unprocessed foods the foundation of your diet. These nutrient-dense choices provide a wide array of vitamins, minerals, and fiber, supporting overall health and well-being.

Monitor Portion Sizes: Pay attention to portion sizes to avoid excessive carbohydrate consumption, even with low-GI foods. Balanced portions help maintain blood sugar stability and support weight management.

Stay Hydrated: Keep hydrated with water and avoid sugary beverages, which can cause rapid blood sugar spikes.

Seek Professional Guidance: Consult with a healthcare professional or a registered dietitian to personalize your GI diet plan, especially if you have specific health concerns or dietary needs.

Remember, the Glycemic Index diet is not about deprivation; rather, it is about making smart food choices that nourish your body and promote optimal health. By following these steps and incorporating low-GI foods into your meals, you can embark on a fulfilling and sustainable journey towards a balanced and healthier lifestyle.

Assessing Your Current Eating Habits

Embarking on a journey towards better health begins with a critical step: assessing your current eating habits. Understanding what you consume daily provides valuable insights into how your diet may be impacting your overall well-being. By taking the time to evaluate your food choices, you can identify areas for improvement and make informed decisions to support your health goals.

Start by keeping a food diary for a few days, documenting everything you eat and drink. Be honest and detailed, noting portion sizes and any snacks consumed between meals. This record will serve as a snapshot of your eating patterns, enabling you to see both strengths and areas that may need adjustment.

Next, examine your food choices for patterns related to the Glycemic Index (GI). Pay attention to the types of carbohydrates you consume, particularly those with high-GI values, such as sugary treats, white bread, and processed snacks. These foods can lead to rapid spikes in blood sugar levels, impacting energy levels and overall well-being.

Consider your overall nutrient intake as well. Are you incorporating enough fruits, vegetables, whole grains, and lean proteins into your meals? Or is your diet heavily reliant on processed and convenience foods? Evaluating your nutrient intake can help you identify areas where you can make healthier choices.

Moreover, be mindful of your portion sizes and eating habits. Are you eating when you're hungry or out of boredom or stress? Are your portion sizes appropriate, or do you find yourself overeating?

As you assess your eating habits, remember that this is not about self-criticism or judgment but rather an opportunity for positive change. Recognize your progress and accomplishments, and be kind to yourself throughout the process.

Once you have a clear understanding of your current eating habits, you can begin making small, sustainable changes to improve your diet. Incorporate more low-GI foods, such as whole grains, fruits, and vegetables, into your meals while reducing high-GI options. Aim for balanced and nutrient-dense meals, and consider seeking guidance from a healthcare professional or a registered dietitian to tailor a personalized plan that aligns with your health goals.

Assessing your current eating habits is an empowering step towards a healthier you. Armed with this knowledge, you can make informed food choices that support your well-being and pave the way for a more balanced and nourishing lifestyle. Remember, each small change adds up, and with patience and commitment, you can create lasting positive changes for your health and happiness.

The Basics of the Glycemic Index Diet

The Glycemic Index (GI) diet is a simple yet powerful approach to eating that focuses on making smart carbohydrate choices to support overall health and well-being. At its core, the GI diet is about understanding how different carbohydrates impact blood sugar levels and choosing foods that have a lower glycemic response.

The GI scale ranks carbohydrates on a scale from 0 to 100 based on how quickly they raise blood sugar levels. Foods with a high GI (70 or above) cause rapid spikes in blood sugar, leading to quick energy bursts followed by crashes. On the other hand, foods with a low GI (55 or below) result in a more gradual and sustained increase in blood sugar, providing steady energy levels and promoting a feeling of fullness.

At the foundation of the GI diet are whole, unprocessed foods that are nutrient-dense and rich in fiber. Non-starchy vegetables, whole grains, legumes, and most fruits are excellent low-GI choices that offer a wide array of vitamins, minerals, and antioxidants. These foods also promote satiety, making it easier to manage hunger and prevent overeating.

In contrast, high-GI foods, such as sugary treats, refined grains, and some processed snacks, should be consumed in moderation. These foods can lead to rapid fluctuations in blood sugar levels and may contribute to weight gain and insulin resistance.

Balancing meals on the GI diet involves combining low-GI carbohydrates with lean proteins and healthy fats. This combination further slows down the digestion and absorption of carbohydrates, promoting better blood sugar control and supporting sustained energy levels.

The GI diet is not a restrictive plan but rather a flexible and sustainable approach to eating. By choosing low-GI foods and prioritizing whole, nutrient-dense options, individuals can nourish their bodies, optimize energy levels, and support overall health.

Incorporating the basics of the Glycemic Index diet into your daily life doesn't require drastic changes; it simply involves making mindful and informed food choices. Gradually replace high-GI foods with low-GI alternatives, experiment with new recipes, and pay attention to how your body responds to different foods.

Remember, the Glycemic Index diet is a tool that can be tailored to suit your individual needs and preferences. By embracing the basics of the GI diet, you can embark on a journey towards a balanced and nourishing way of eating that promotes overall health and vitality.

Creating a Balanced Meal Plan

Crafting a balanced meal plan is a fundamental aspect of promoting overall health and well-being. A well-balanced diet provides the body with essential nutrients, supports energy levels, and helps maintain stable blood sugar levels. Whether you are following the Glycemic Index (GI) diet or simply striving for a healthier lifestyle, a balanced meal plan is key to nourishing your body and optimizing your daily performance.

Start by incorporating a variety of food groups into your meals. Aim to include a mix of non-starchy vegetables, whole grains, lean proteins, and healthy fats in each meal. Vegetables provide a wealth of vitamins, minerals, and fiber, while whole grains offer sustained energy and additional fiber to support digestive health. Lean proteins, such as poultry, fish, tofu, or legumes, supply essential amino acids for muscle repair and overall body function. Healthy fats, found in avocados, nuts, seeds, and olive oil, are crucial for brain health and nutrient absorption.

When planning your meals, consider the Glycemic Index of the foods you choose. Strive to incorporate more low-GI foods that provide a steady source of energy and help regulate blood sugar levels. Pair low-GI carbohydrates with proteins and healthy fats to further slow down the digestion process and enhance the overall nutritional value of your meals.

Portion control is another essential aspect of a balanced meal plan. Be mindful of serving sizes to avoid overeating and unnecessary calorie consumption. Listen to your body's hunger and fullness cues to ensure you are eating in tune with your body's needs.

Meal planning can be a fun and creative process. Experiment with new recipes and flavors, and don't be afraid to try different cuisines or ingredients. Keep your meals diverse and enjoyable to sustain your commitment to a balanced diet.

Lastly, stay hydrated throughout the day by drinking plenty of water. Hydration is essential for maintaining bodily functions and can help you distinguish between hunger and thirst cues.

A balanced meal plan not only nourishes your body with optimal nutrition but also sets the stage for a lifetime of healthy eating habits. Whether your goal is to manage blood sugar levels or enhance overall well-being, creating a balanced meal plan provides the foundation for a balanced and nourishing lifestyle. Remember, small changes can yield significant results, and every step towards a more balanced diet is a step towards a healthier you.

Smart Carbohydrate Choices

When it comes to carbohydrate choices, not all foods are created equal. Making smart carbohydrate choices is a fundamental aspect of maintaining stable blood sugar levels, promoting sustained energy, and supporting overall health. Whether you are following the Glycemic Index (GI) diet or simply striving for a balanced and nourishing lifestyle, opting for nutrient-dense carbohydrates can make a significant difference in your well-being.

Whole grains are a fantastic example of smart carbohydrate choices. They are rich in fiber, vitamins, and minerals, providing sustained energy and promoting digestive health. Incorporate whole grains such as quinoa, brown rice, and oats into your meals to enjoy their nutritional benefits.

Non-starchy vegetables are another excellent option for smart carbohydrate choices. Low in calories and high in fiber, vitamins, and antioxidants, vegetables like leafy greens, broccoli, and bell peppers are essential for a well-rounded diet. They promote satiety, aid in weight management, and contribute to overall well-being.

Legumes, such as lentils, chickpeas, and black beans, are excellent sources of protein and complex carbohydrates. They have a low glycemic response, making them ideal choices for stable blood sugar levels and sustained energy.

Fruits are natural sources of carbohydrates that offer a plethora of vitamins, minerals, and fiber. Opt for whole fruits rather than fruit juices or processed fruit products to maximize their nutritional benefits and minimize the glycemic impact.

Sweet potatoes are a nutrient-dense and flavorful carbohydrate option. They are rich in vitamins A and C, potassium, and fiber, making them an excellent choice for a balanced meal.

When choosing carbohydrates, be mindful of processed and refined options that can lead to rapid spikes in blood sugar levels. Limit your intake of sugary treats, pastries, and white bread, which have higher glycemic responses and provide empty calories.

Remember, smart carbohydrate choices are not about restriction but about making conscious decisions that support your health and well-being. By incorporating nutrient-dense carbohydrates into your diet, you can nourish your body with essential nutrients, promote sustained energy, and enjoy the benefits of a balanced and nourishing lifestyle.

Chapter 2

Low-GI Breakfast Recipes

Welcome to a collection of delightful Low-GI Breakfast Recipes designed to kickstart your day with a burst of sustained energy and balanced nutrition. The Glycemic Index (GI) diet focuses on making smart carbohydrate choices to support stable blood sugar levels, and breakfast is the perfect opportunity to set the tone for a day of vitality and well-being.

This carefully curated assortment of Low-GI Breakfast Recipes showcases the harmonious blend of taste and health. From nourishing overnight oats infused with the sweetness of berries to protein-packed veggie egg muffins that elevate your morning routine, these recipes offer a diverse array of options to suit every palate.

Start your day with a delectable quinoa breakfast bowl, lusciously cooked in almond milk and adorned with sliced bananas and toasted almonds. Or indulge in the comforting goodness of whole grain pancakes, drizzled with pure maple syrup and crowned with fresh fruit.

These Low-GI Breakfast Recipes cater to those seeking sustained energy, improved satiety, and balanced blood sugar levels. Whether you follow the Glycemic Index diet or simply embrace a healthier lifestyle, these recipes are the perfect embodiment of nourishing your body with love and care.

Join us on this culinary journey as we explore the world of Low-GI Breakfast Recipes that will leave you feeling revitalized and ready to take on the day with a smile. Your mornings will never be the same again as you savor each bite, knowing that you are nourishing your body with the finest ingredients for a vibrant and thriving life.

Berry and Almond Overnight Oats

Classic Mixed Berry Overnight Oats:

Ingredients:

- 1/2 cup rolled oats
- 1 cup almond milk
- 1 tablespoon chia seeds
- 1 tablespoon almond butter
- 1 teaspoon pure maple syrup
- 1/2 cup mixed berries (strawberries, blueberries, and raspberries)

Preparation:

In a mason jar or container, combine rolled oats, almond milk, chia seeds, almond butter, and maple syrup.Stir well to ensure everything is evenly mixed.

Add the mixed berries on top and gently press them into the oat mixture.Seal the jar and refrigerate overnight. In the morning, give it a quick stir and enjoy your berry and almond-infused breakfast.

Tropical Berry and Almond Overnight Oats:

Ingredients:

- 1/2 cup rolled oats
- 1 cup coconut milk
- 1 tablespoon shredded coconut
- 1 tablespoon almond butter
- 1 teaspoon honey or agave syrup
- 1/2 cup mixed berries (strawberries, blackberries, and kiwi slices)

Preparation:

Combine rolled oats, coconut milk, shredded coconut, almond butter, and sweetener of your choice in a jar or container. Mix well until all ingredients are thoroughly combined. Top with the mixed berries and kiwi slices. Seal the jar and refrigerate overnight. Wake up to a tropical delight and savor the tropical flavors of this berry and almond-infused overnight oats.

Raspberry Almond Delight Overnight Oats:

Ingredients:

- 1/2 cup rolled oats
- 1 cup almond milk
- 1 tablespoon almond butter
- 1 tablespoon raspberry jam
- 1/4 cup fresh raspberries
- 1 tablespoon sliced almonds

Preparation:

In a jar or container, combine rolled oats, almond milk, almond butter, and raspberry jam. Stir until well incorporated. Add fresh raspberries and sliced almonds on top. Seal the jar and refrigerate overnight. Wake up to a delightful combination of raspberries and almonds in your creamy overnight oats.

Blueberry Bliss Overnight Oats:

Ingredients:

- 1/2 cup rolled oats
- 1 cup almond milk
- 1 tablespoon almond butter
- 1 tablespoon honey or agave syrup

- 1/2 cup fresh blueberries
- 1 tablespoon chopped almonds

Preparation:

Combine rolled oats, almond milk, almond butter, and sweetener in a jar or container. Mix until everything is well combined. Add fresh blueberries and chopped almonds on top. Seal the jar and refrigerate overnight. Wake up to a burst of blueberry bliss in your almond-infused overnight oats.

Blackberry and Almond Crunch Overnight Oats:

Ingredients:

- 1/2 cup rolled oats
- 1 cup almond milk
- 1 tablespoon almond butter
- 1 tablespoon honey or agave syrup
- 1/2 cup fresh blackberries
- 1 tablespoon granola

Preparation:

In a jar or container, combine rolled oats, almond milk, almond butter, and sweetener. Stir until all ingredients are incorporated. Top with fresh blackberries and a sprinkle of granola for added crunch. Seal the jar and refrigerate overnight. Wake up to a delightful and crunchy blackberry and almond-flavored breakfast.

Enjoy these 100% unique and nutritious Berry and Almond Overnight Oats recipes, perfect for a satisfying and wholesome morning meal that energizes you for the day ahead.

Vegetable Egg Muffins

Spinach and Feta Egg Muffins:

Ingredients:

- 6 large eggs
- 1 cup baby spinach, chopped
- 1/2 cup crumbled feta cheese
- 1/4 cup diced red bell pepper
- 1/4 cup diced red onion
- 1 teaspoon olive oil
- Salt and pepper to taste

Preparation:

Preheat the oven to 350°F (175°C) and grease a muffin tin. In a skillet, heat olive oil over medium heat and sauté the diced red bell pepper and red onion until softened. In a mixing bowl, beat the eggs and season with salt and pepper. Stir in the sautéed vegetables, chopped spinach, and crumbled feta cheese. Pour the mixture evenly into the muffin tin. Bake for 18-20 minutes or until the egg muffins are set and lightly golden. Let them cool slightly before serving.

Mushroom and Swiss Egg Muffins:

Ingredients:

- 6 large eggs
- 1 cup sliced mushrooms
- 1/2 cup shredded Swiss cheese
- 2 tablespoons chopped fresh parsley
- 1 tablespoon olive oil
- Salt and pepper to taste

Preparation:

Preheat the oven to 350°F (175°C) and grease a muffin tin. In a skillet, heat olive oil over medium heat and sauté the sliced mushrooms until tender. In a mixing bowl, beat the eggs and season with salt and pepper. Stir in the sautéed mushrooms, shredded Swiss cheese, and chopped parsley. Pour the mixture evenly into the muffin tin. Bake for 18-20 minutes or until the egg muffins are set and the cheese is melted. Let them cool slightly before serving.

Tomato, Basil, and Mozzarella Egg Muffins:

Ingredients:

- 6 large eggs
- 1 cup cherry tomatoes, halved
- 1/2 cup fresh mozzarella, diced
- 1/4 cup chopped fresh basil
- 1 tablespoon olive oil
- Salt and pepper to taste

Preparation:

Preheat the oven to 350°F (175°C) and grease a muffin tin. In a skillet, heat olive oil over medium heat and sauté the halved cherry tomatoes until softened. In a mixing bowl, beat the eggs and season with salt and pepper. Stir in the sautéed cherry tomatoes, diced mozzarella, and chopped basil. Pour the mixture evenly into the muffin tin. Bake for 18-20 minutes or until the egg muffins are set and lightly golden. Let them cool slightly before serving.

Broccoli and Cheddar Egg Muffins:

Ingredients:

- 6 large eggs
- 1 cup chopped broccoli florets
- 1/2 cup shredded cheddar cheese
- 1/4 cup diced red bell pepper

- 1 tablespoon olive oil
- Salt and pepper to taste

Preparation:

Preheat the oven to 350°F (175°C) and grease a muffin tin. In a skillet, heat olive oil over medium heat and sauté the chopped broccoli florets and diced red bell pepper until tender. In a mixing bowl, beat the eggs and season with salt and pepper. Stir in the sautéed broccoli and red bell pepper, and shredded cheddar cheese. Pour the mixture evenly into the muffin tin. Bake for 18-20 minutes or until the egg muffins are set and the cheese is melted. Let them cool slightly before serving.

Zucchini and Parmesan Egg Muffins:

Ingredients:

- 6 large eggs
- 1 cup grated zucchini
- 1/2 cup grated Parmesan cheese
- 2 tablespoons chopped fresh basil
- 1 tablespoon olive oil
- Salt and pepper to taste

Preparation:

Preheat the oven to 350°F (175°C) and grease a muffin tin. In a skillet, heat olive oil over medium heat and sauté the grated zucchini until softened. In a mixing bowl, beat the eggs and season with salt and pepper. Stir in the sautéed zucchini, grated Parmesan cheese, and chopped basil. Pour the mixture evenly into the muffin tin. Bake for 18-20 minutes or until the egg muffins are set and lightly golden. Let them cool slightly before serving.

Enjoy these 100% unique and delicious Vegetable Egg Muffins recipes, perfect for a quick and nutritious breakfast or snack on the go. Customize the ingredients to your taste and embrace the convenience of these flavorful egg muffins.

Quinoa and Blueberry Breakfast Bowl

Classic Quinoa Blueberry Breakfast Bowl:

Ingredients:

- 1 cup cooked quinoa
- 1/2 cup fresh blueberries
- 2 tablespoons chopped almonds
- 1 tablespoon honey
- 1/4 teaspoon ground cinnamon

Preparation:

 In a bowl, combine the cooked quinoa, fresh blueberries, and chopped almonds. Drizzle with honey and sprinkle ground cinnamon on top. Mix everything together until well combined. Enjoy this delightful and nutritious blueberry breakfast bowl to start your day on a healthy note.

Tropical Quinoa Blueberry Breakfast Bowl:

Ingredients:

- 1 cup cooked quinoa
- 1/2 cup fresh blueberries
- 1/2 cup diced mango
- 2 tablespoons shredded coconut
- 1 tablespoon agave syrup or maple syrup

Preparation:

In a bowl, mix the cooked quinoa, fresh blueberries, diced mango, and shredded coconut. Drizzle with agave syrup or maple syrup for a touch of sweetness. Stir well until all the ingredients are evenly distributed. Savor the tropical flavors of this refreshing quinoa blueberry breakfast bowl.

Protein-Packed Quinoa Blueberry Breakfast Bowl:

Ingredients:

- 1 cup cooked quinoa
- 1/2 cup fresh blueberries
- 1/4 cup sliced almonds
- 2 tablespoons hemp seeds
- 1 tablespoon almond butter
- 1 teaspoon vanilla extract

Preparation: I

n a bowl, combine the cooked quinoa, fresh blueberries, sliced almonds, and hemp seeds. Drizzle with almond butter and add vanilla extract for flavor. Mix everything together until the ingredients are well incorporated. This protein-packed quinoa blueberry breakfast bowl will keep you fueled and satisfied throughout the morning.

Creamy Quinoa Blueberry Breakfast Bowl:

Ingredients:

- 1 cup cooked quinoa
- 1/2 cup fresh blueberries
- 1/4 cup Greek yogurt
- 1 tablespoon honey
- 1/2 teaspoon lemon zest

Preparation:

In a bowl, mix the cooked quinoa, fresh blueberries, Greek yogurt, honey, and lemon zest. Stir until the ingredients are thoroughly combined and the yogurt coats the quinoa and blueberries. Revel in the creamy and tangy goodness of this delightful quinoa blueberry breakfast bowl.

Chocolaty Quinoa Blueberry Breakfast Bowl:

Ingredients:

- 1 cup cooked quinoa
- 1/2 cup fresh blueberries
- 2 tablespoons dark chocolate chips
- 1 tablespoon unsweetened cocoa powder
- 1 tablespoon maple syrup

Preparation:

In a bowl, combine the cooked quinoa, fresh blueberries, dark chocolate chips, cocoa powder, and maple syrup. Mix everything together until the chocolate chips and cocoa powder coat the quinoa and blueberries. Indulge in the decadence of this chocolaty quinoa blueberry breakfast bowl, perfect for satisfying your sweet cravings in a wholesome way.

Enjoy these 100% unique and delicious Quinoa and Blueberry Breakfast Bowl recipes, packed with nutrients and bursting with flavor. Customize the ingredients to your liking and embrace the versatility of quinoa and blueberries in creating a nourishing and delightful morning meal.

Chapter 3

Wholesome Lunch Ideas

Welcome to a world of nourishing and delightful Wholesome Lunch Ideas that will invigorate your midday meals with an abundance of flavors, nutrients, and satisfaction. Whether you're seeking to maintain a healthy lifestyle, enhance productivity, or simply indulge in delicious and wholesome food, these lunch ideas are here to inspire and nourish you.

In our fast-paced lives, taking a moment to enjoy a well-balanced lunch is a gift we can give ourselves. Wholesome lunch choices not only fuel our bodies but also contribute to overall well-being, ensuring we stay energized and focused throughout the day. From nutrient-packed salads and hearty soups to mouthwatering wraps and grain bowls, there's something for every palate and dietary preference.

Each of these Wholesome Lunch Ideas celebrates the beauty of fresh, whole ingredients that promote physical and mental wellness. The recipes are carefully curated to strike a harmonious balance between taste and nutrition, making lunchtime an enjoyable and health-enhancing experience.

Whether you're a busy professional, a student, or a home cook, these lunch ideas are designed to fit seamlessly into your daily routine. So, bid farewell to bland and mundane lunches and embrace the array of colors, flavors, and textures that these recipes offer.

Join us on this journey of culinary exploration as we unlock the potential of wholesome lunchtime indulgence. Let's revel in the joy of nourishing our bodies and elevating our lunchtime experience with these 100% unique and inspiring Wholesome Lunch Ideas. Your taste buds and well-being will thank you for it!

Mediterranean Chickpea Salad

Classic Mediterranean Chickpea Salad:

Ingredients:

- 1 can (15 oz) chickpeas, drained and rinsed
- 1 cup cherry tomatoes, halved
- 1 cucumber, diced
- 1/4 cup Kalamata olives, pitted and halved
- 1/4 cup red onion, thinly sliced
- 1/4 cup crumbled feta cheese
- 2 tablespoons fresh lemon juice
- 2 tablespoons extra-virgin olive oil
- 2 tablespoons chopped fresh parsley
- Salt and pepper to taste

Preparation:

In a large bowl, combine chickpeas, cherry tomatoes, cucumber, Kalamata olives, red onion, and crumbled feta cheese. In a separate small bowl, whisk together lemon juice, olive oil, chopped parsley, salt, and pepper. Pour the dressing over the salad and toss gently to coat all the ingredients. Serve immediately or refrigerate for a refreshing and satisfying Mediterranean-inspired lunch.

Quinoa Mediterranean Chickpea Salad:

Ingredients:

- 1 cup cooked quinoa
- 1 can (15 oz) chickpeas, drained and rinsed
- 1/2 cup diced cucumber
- 1/2 cup diced red bell pepper
- 1/4 cup sliced black olives
- 1/4 cup crumbled feta cheese
- 2 tablespoons red wine vinegar
- 2 tablespoons extra-virgin olive oil
- 1 tablespoon chopped fresh oregano
- Salt and pepper to taste

Preparation:

In a large bowl, combine cooked quinoa, chickpeas, cucumber, red bell pepper, black olives, and crumbled feta cheese. In a small bowl, whisk together red wine vinegar, olive oil, chopped oregano, salt, and pepper. Drizzle the dressing over the salad and toss gently until well combined. Enjoy this hearty and wholesome Mediterranean chickpea salad with the goodness of quinoa.

Roasted Vegetable Mediterranean Chickpea Salad:

Ingredients:

- 1 can (15 oz) chickpeas, drained and rinsed
- 1 cup cherry tomatoes
- 1 zucchini, diced
- 1 red bell pepper, diced
- 1 tablespoon olive oil
- 1 teaspoon ground cumin
- 1/2 teaspoon paprika
- 1/4 teaspoon garlic powder
- Salt and pepper to taste
- 2 tablespoons chopped fresh basil

Preparation:

Preheat the oven to 400°F (200°C). In a baking sheet, toss the chickpeas, cherry tomatoes, diced zucchini, and red bell pepper with olive oil, ground cumin, paprika, garlic powder, salt, and pepper. Roast in the oven for 20-25 minutes until the vegetables are tender and slightly caramelized. Remove from the oven and let them cool slightly. Transfer the roasted vegetables and chickpeas to a bowl and sprinkle with chopped fresh basil. This Mediterranean chickpea salad with roasted vegetables is bursting with flavor and texture.

Greek-Inspired Mediterranean Chickpea Salad:

Ingredients:

- 1 can (15 oz) chickpeas, drained and rinsed
- 1 cup cucumber, diced
- 1/2 cup cherry tomatoes, halved
- 1/4 cup red onion, thinly sliced
- 1/4 cup Kalamata olives, pitted and halved
- 1/4 cup crumbled feta cheese
- 2 tablespoons chopped fresh dill
- 2 tablespoons fresh lemon juice
- 2 tablespoons extra-virgin olive oil
- Salt and pepper to taste

Preparation:

In a large bowl, combine chickpeas, cucumber, cherry tomatoes, red onion, Kalamata olives, and crumbled feta cheese. In a separate small bowl, whisk together fresh lemon juice, olive oil, chopped dill, salt, and pepper. Pour the dressing over the salad and toss gently until all the ingredients are well coated. Embrace the flavors of Greece with this tangy and savory Mediterranean chickpea salad.

Spinach and Chickpea Mediterranean Salad:

Ingredients:

- 1 can (15 oz) chickpeas, drained and rinsed
- 2 cups fresh baby spinach leaves
- 1/4 cup sun-dried tomatoes, chopped
- 1/4 cup toasted pine nuts
- 2 tablespoons balsamic vinegar
- 2 tablespoons extra-virgin olive oil
- 1 tablespoon honey or maple syrup
- Salt and pepper to taste

Preparation:

In a large bowl, combine chickpeas, fresh baby spinach leaves, chopped sun-dried tomatoes, and toasted pine nuts. In a separate small bowl, whisk together balsamic vinegar, olive oil, honey (or maple syrup), salt, and pepper. Drizzle the dressing over the salad and toss gently until well combined. This spinach and chickpea Mediterranean salad offers a delightful mix of textures and flavors.

Enjoy these 100% unique and wholesome Mediterranean Chickpea Salad recipes, each bursting with the vibrant flavors of the Mediterranean region.

These salads are not only delicious but also packed with essential nutrients to nourish your body and delight your taste buds. Whether you choose to enjoy them as a refreshing lunch or a satisfying side, these chickpea salads are a celebration of fresh and wholesome ingredients.

Grilled Chicken and Vegetable Skewers

Classic Grilled Chicken and Vegetable Skewers:

Ingredients:

- 2 boneless, skinless chicken breasts, cut into chunks
- 1 red bell pepper, cut into chunks
- 1 green bell pepper, cut into chunks
- 1 red onion, cut into chunks
- 8 cherry tomatoes
- 2 tablespoons olive oil
- 2 tablespoons lemon juice
- 2 cloves garlic, minced
- 1 teaspoon dried oregano
- Salt and pepper to taste

Preparation:

In a bowl, combine olive oil, lemon juice, minced garlic, dried oregano, salt, and pepper to create the marinade. Add the chicken chunks to the marinade and let it marinate for at least 30 minutes. Thread the marinated chicken chunks onto skewers, alternating with the bell peppers, red onion, and cherry tomatoes. Preheat the grill to medium-high heat and cook the skewers for about 10-12 minutes, turning occasionally, until the chicken is cooked through and the vegetables are slightly charred. Serve these classic grilled chicken and vegetable skewers with your favorite dipping sauce or over a bed of rice.

Teriyaki Chicken and Pineapple Skewers:

Ingredients:

- 2 boneless, skinless chicken breasts, cut into chunks
- 1 cup pineapple chunks
- 1 red bell pepper, cut into chunks
- 1 green bell pepper, cut into chunks
- 1 red onion, cut into chunks
- 1/4 cup teriyaki sauce
- 2 tablespoons soy sauce
- 2 tablespoons honey
- 1 tablespoon sesame oil
- Salt and pepper to taste

Preparation:

In a bowl, whisk together teriyaki sauce, soy sauce, honey, sesame oil, salt, and pepper to create the marinade. Add the chicken chunks to the marinade and let it marinate for about 1 hour. Thread the marinated chicken chunks onto skewers, alternating with pineapple chunks, bell peppers, and red onion. Preheat the grill to medium-high heat and cook the skewers for about 10-12 minutes, turning occasionally, until the chicken is cooked through and the vegetables are slightly charred. Serve these teriyaki chicken and pineapple skewers with steamed rice or a side of stir-fried vegetables.

Lemon Herb Chicken and Zucchini Skewers:

Ingredients:

- 2 boneless, skinless chicken breasts, cut into chunks
- 2 zucchini, sliced into thick rounds
- 1 lemon, sliced
- 2 tablespoons olive oil
- 2 cloves garlic, minced
- 1 tablespoon chopped fresh herbs (such as rosemary, thyme, or basil)
- Salt and pepper to taste

Preparation:

In a bowl, combine olive oil, minced garlic, chopped fresh herbs, salt, and pepper to create the marinade. Add the chicken chunks to the marinade and let it marinate for about 30 minutes. Thread the marinated chicken chunks onto skewers, alternating with zucchini slices and lemon slices. Preheat the grill to medium-high heat and cook the skewers for about 10-12 minutes, turning occasionally, until the chicken is cooked through and the zucchini is tender. Squeeze some fresh lemon juice over the skewers before serving.

Spicy Cajun Chicken and Pepper Skewers:

Ingredients:

- 2 boneless, skinless chicken breasts, cut into chunks
- 1 red bell pepper, cut into chunks
- 1 yellow bell pepper, cut into chunks
- 1 green bell pepper, cut into chunks
- 2 tablespoons olive oil
- 1 tablespoon Cajun seasoning
- 1 teaspoon paprika
- 1/2 teaspoon garlic powder
- Salt and pepper to taste

Preparation:

In a bowl, combine olive oil, Cajun seasoning, paprika, garlic powder, salt, and pepper to create the marinade. Add the chicken chunks to the marinade and let it marinate for at least 30 minutes. Thread the marinated chicken chunks onto skewers, alternating with the bell pepper chunks. Preheat the grill to medium-high heat and cook the skewers for about 10-12 minutes, turning occasionally, until the chicken is cooked through and the peppers are slightly charred. Serve these spicy Cajun chicken and pepper skewers with a side of rice or a crisp green salad.

Honey Mustard Chicken and Mushroom Skewers:

Ingredients:

- 2 boneless, skinless chicken breasts, cut into chunks
- 8-10 button mushrooms
- 1 red onion, cut into chunks
- 2 tablespoons Dijon mustard
- 2 tablespoons honey
- 1 tablespoon apple cider vinegar
- 1 tablespoon olive oil
- Salt and pepper to taste

Preparation:

In a bowl, whisk together Dijon mustard, honey, apple cider vinegar, olive oil, salt, and pepper to create the marinade. Add the chicken chunks to the marinade and let it marinate for about 1 hour. Thread the marinated chicken chunks onto skewers, alternating with mushrooms and red onion chunks. Preheat the grill to medium-high heat and cook the skewers for about 10-12 minutes, turning occasionally, until the chicken is cooked through and the mushrooms are tender. Drizzle any remaining marinade over the skewers before serving.

Enjoy these 100% unique and flavorful Grilled Chicken and Vegetable Skewer recipes. They are versatile, easy to prepare, and perfect for summer grilling or any time you crave a delicious and healthy meal. Get creative with your choice of vegetables and seasonings to customize these skewers to your taste preferences. Whether you're hosting a backyard barbecue or enjoying a casual weeknight dinner, these skewers will surely impress with their tantalizing flavors and juicy textures.

Spinach and Feta Stuffed Portobello Mushrooms

Classic Spinach and Feta Stuffed Portobello Mushrooms:

Ingredients:

- 5 large Portobello mushrooms, stems removed
- 2 cups fresh spinach, chopped
- 1 cup crumbled feta cheese
- 1/4 cup diced red onion
- 2 cloves garlic, minced
- 2 tablespoons olive oil
- 1 tablespoon balsamic vinegar
- Salt and pepper to taste

Preparation:

Preheat the oven to 375°F (190°C). In a skillet, heat the olive oil over medium heat and sauté the minced garlic and diced red onion until softened. Add the chopped spinach and cook until wilted. Remove the skillet from the heat and stir in the crumbled feta cheese. Season the mixture with salt and pepper to taste. Place the Portobello mushrooms on a baking sheet and drizzle with balsamic vinegar. Stuff each mushroom with the spinach and feta mixture. Bake in the preheated oven for about 15-20 minutes until the mushrooms are tender and the filling is golden and bubbly.

Mediterranean Quinoa Spinach and Feta Stuffed Portobello Mushrooms:

Ingredients:

- 5 large Portobello mushrooms, stems removed
- 1 cup cooked quinoa
- 1 cup fresh baby spinach, chopped
- 1/2 cup crumbled feta cheese
- 1/4 cup sun-dried tomatoes, chopped
- 2 tablespoons chopped fresh basil
- 1 tablespoon lemon juice
- 2 tablespoons olive oil
- Salt and pepper to taste

Preparation:

Preheat the oven to 375°F (190°C). In a bowl, combine cooked quinoa, chopped baby spinach, crumbled feta cheese, chopped sun-dried tomatoes, chopped fresh basil, lemon juice, olive oil, salt, and pepper. Place the Portobello mushrooms on a baking sheet and drizzle with olive oil. Stuff each mushroom with the quinoa mixture. Bake in the preheated oven for about 15-20 minutes until the mushrooms are tender and the filling is heated through.

Spinach and Feta Stuffed Portobello Mushrooms with Pesto:

Ingredients:

- 5 large Portobello mushrooms, stems removed
- 2 cups fresh baby spinach, chopped
- 1 cup crumbled feta cheese
- 1/4 cup toasted pine nuts
- 2 tablespoons store-bought or homemade pesto
- 2 tablespoons olive oil
- Salt and pepper to taste

Preparation:

Preheat the oven to 375°F (190°C). In a skillet, heat the olive oil over medium heat and sauté the chopped baby spinach until wilted. Remove the skillet from the heat and stir in the crumbled feta cheese and toasted pine nuts. Season the mixture with salt and pepper to taste. Place the Portobello mushrooms on a baking sheet and drizzle with olive oil. Spread a thin layer of pesto on the inside of each mushroom cap. Stuff each mushroom with the spinach and feta mixture. Bake in the preheated oven for about 15-20 minutes until the mushrooms are tender and the filling is heated through.

Greek-Inspired Spinach and Feta Stuffed Portobello Mushrooms:

Ingredients:

- 5 large Portobello mushrooms, stems removed
- 2 cups fresh baby spinach, chopped
- 1 cup crumbled feta cheese
- 1/4 cup pitted Kalamata olives, chopped
- 1/4 cup diced red onion
- 2 tablespoons chopped fresh dill
- 2 tablespoons lemon juice
- 2 tablespoons olive oil
- Salt and pepper to taste

Preparation:

Preheat the oven to 375°F (190°C). In a skillet, heat the olive oil over medium heat and sauté the chopped baby spinach until wilted. Remove the skillet from the heat and stir in the crumbled feta cheese, chopped Kalamata olives, diced red onion, chopped fresh dill, lemon juice, salt, and pepper. Place the Portobello mushrooms on a baking sheet and drizzle with olive oil. Stuff each mushroom with the spinach and feta mixture. Bake in the preheated oven for about 15-20 minutes until the mushrooms are tender and the filling is heated through.

Spinach and Feta Stuffed Portobello Mushrooms with Breadcrumbs:

Ingredients:

- 5 large Portobello mushrooms, stems removed
- 2 cups fresh baby spinach, chopped
- 1 cup crumbled feta cheese
- 1/4 cup breadcrumbs
- 2 tablespoons chopped fresh parsley
- 1 tablespoon lemon zest
- 2 tablespoons olive oil
- Salt and pepper to taste

Preparation:

Preheat the oven to 375°F (190°C). In a skillet, heat the olive oil over medium heat and sauté the chopped baby spinach until wilted. Remove the skillet from the heat and stir in the crumbled feta cheese, breadcrumbs, chopped fresh parsley, lemon zest, salt, and pepper. Place the Portobello mushrooms on a baking sheet and drizzle with olive oil. Stuff each mushroom with the spinach and feta mixture. Bake in the preheated oven for about 15-20 minutes until the mushrooms are tender and the filling is heated through.

Enjoy these 100% unique and flavorful Spinach and Feta Stuffed Portobello Mushrooms recipes. Each one is a perfect blend of wholesome ingredients and delightful flavors, making them a delicious and satisfying option for a vegetarian main course or a hearty side dish. Experiment with different combinations of herbs, seasonings, and toppings to create your personalized version of these stuffed mushrooms. Whether served as an appetizer or a main course, these stuffed Portobello mushrooms are sure to impress your guests and satisfy your taste buds.

Chapter 4

Nutritious Dinner Options

Welcome to the world of Nutritious Dinner Options, where health and flavor come together to create delightful and wholesome meals for you and your loved ones. In today's fast-paced world, finding time to prepare nourishing dinners can be a challenge, but it doesn't have to be. This cookbook aims to inspire you with a collection of delectable and nutrient-packed dinner recipes that are easy to make and will leave you feeling energized and satisfied.

We understand that a well-balanced dinner is crucial for overall health and well-being. Our recipes are carefully curated to incorporate a variety of fresh, seasonal ingredients that provide essential nutrients, vitamins, and minerals. Whether you're a seasoned home cook or a beginner, these recipes are designed to be approachable and enjoyable for everyone.

From flavorful plant-based options that celebrate the bounties of nature to protein-rich dishes that will please even the most discerning carnivores, this cookbook offers a diverse range of dinner ideas that cater to different dietary preferences and restrictions.

Embrace the joy of cooking as you explore these nutritious dinner options, each dish crafted with love and attention to ensure a harmonious blend of taste and nutrition. So, let's embark on a culinary journey that prioritizes health without compromising on flavor. Get ready to savor every bite and nourish your body with the goodness it deserves!

Baked Cod with Roasted Vegetables

Lemon Herb Baked Cod with Roasted Asparagus and Cherry Tomatoes:

Ingredients:

- 4 cod fillets
- 1 bunch asparagus, trimmed
- 1 cup cherry tomatoes
- 2 tablespoons olive oil
- 2 cloves garlic, minced
- 1 tablespoon chopped fresh parsley
- 1 tablespoon chopped fresh thyme
- Zest of 1 lemon
- Salt and pepper to taste

Preparation:

Preheat the oven to 400°F (200°C). In a large baking dish, place the cod fillets and drizzle with olive oil. Sprinkle minced garlic, chopped parsley, chopped thyme, and lemon zest over the fish. Season with salt and pepper. Toss the trimmed asparagus and cherry tomatoes with olive oil, salt, and pepper, and arrange them around the cod fillets in the baking dish. Bake in the preheated oven for about 15-20 minutes or until the cod is cooked through and flakes easily with a fork. The roasted vegetables should be tender and slightly charred. Serve this lemon herb baked cod with roasted asparagus and cherry tomatoes for a light and flavorful dinner.

Mediterranean Baked Cod with Roasted Bell Peppers and Olives:

Ingredients:

- 4 cod fillets
- 2 bell peppers (red, yellow, or orange), sliced
- 1 cup cherry tomatoes
- 1/2 cup pitted Kalamata olives
- 2 tablespoons olive oil
- 2 tablespoons balsamic vinegar
- 1 teaspoon dried oregano
- Salt and pepper to taste

Preparation:

Preheat the oven to 400°F (200°C). Place the cod fillets in a baking dish and drizzle with olive oil and balsamic vinegar. Sprinkle dried oregano, salt, and pepper over the fish. Toss the sliced bell peppers, cherry tomatoes, and Kalamata olives with olive oil, salt, and pepper. Arrange them around the cod fillets in the baking dish. Bake in the preheated oven for about 15-20 minutes or until the cod is cooked through. The roasted bell peppers and olives will add a burst of Mediterranean flavors to this delicious baked cod dish.

Pesto Crusted Baked Cod with Roasted Brussels Sprouts:

Ingredients:

- 4 cod fillets
- 1 cup fresh basil leaves
- 1/4 cup grated Parmesan cheese
- 1/4 cup pine nuts
- 2 cloves garlic
- 1/4 cup olive oil
- 1 pound Brussels sprouts, halved
- 2 tablespoons balsamic vinegar
- Salt and pepper to taste

Preparation:

Preheat the oven to 400°F (200°C). In a food processor, blend the basil leaves, grated Parmesan cheese, pine nuts, garlic, and olive oil to make the pesto. Spread the pesto mixture over the top of each cod fillet. Place the coated cod fillets in a baking dish. Toss the halved Brussels sprouts with olive oil, balsamic vinegar, salt, and pepper. Arrange them around the cod fillets in the baking dish. Bake in the preheated oven for about 15-20 minutes or until the cod is cooked through and the Brussels sprouts are tender and caramelized.

Dijon Mustard and Herb Baked Cod with Roasted Carrots and Potatoes:

Ingredients:

- 4 cod fillets
- 2 tablespoons Dijon mustard
- 1 tablespoon olive oil
- 1 teaspoon dried thyme
- 1 teaspoon dried rosemary
- 1 pound baby carrots
- 1 pound baby potatoes, halved
- 2 cloves garlic, minced
- Salt and pepper to taste

Preparation:

Preheat the oven to 400°F (200°C). In a small bowl, mix Dijon mustard, olive oil, dried thyme, dried rosemary, minced garlic, salt, and pepper. Spread the Dijon mustard mixture over the top of each cod fillet. Place the coated cod fillets in a baking dish. Toss the baby carrots and halved baby potatoes with olive oil, salt, and pepper. Arrange them around the cod fillets in the baking dish. Bake in the preheated oven for about 15-20 minutes or until the cod is cooked through and the vegetables are tender and golden.

Lemon Garlic Butter Baked Cod with Roasted Broccoli:

Ingredients:

- 4 cod fillets
- 4 tablespoons unsalted butter, melted
- Juice of 1 lemon
- 2 cloves garlic, minced
- 1 tablespoon chopped fresh parsley
- 1 pound broccoli florets
- 2 tablespoons olive oil
- Salt and pepper to taste

Preparation:

Preheat the oven to 400°F (200°C). In a small bowl, mix melted butter, lemon juice, minced garlic, chopped parsley, salt, and pepper. Drizzle the lemon garlic butter mixture over the top of each cod fillet. Place the coated cod fillets in a baking dish. Toss the broccoli florets with olive oil, salt, and pepper. Arrange them around the cod fillets in the baking dish. Bake in the preheated oven for about 15-20 minutes or until the cod is cooked through and the broccoli is tender and slightly crispy.

Enjoy these 100% unique and mouthwatering Baked Cod with Roasted Vegetables recipes. Each dish showcases the natural flavors of the ingredients and offers a delightful combination of textures and tastes. Whether you're looking for a light and zesty Mediterranean twist or a comforting and hearty meal, these recipes will surely become a hit at your dinner table. Get ready to savor the goodness of wholesome ingredients and elevate your dining experience with these delectable baked cod dishes.

Turkey Meatballs with Zucchini Noodles

Classic Turkey Meatballs with Zucchini Noodles:

Ingredients:

- 1 pound ground turkey
- 1/2 cup breadcrumbs
- 1/4 cup grated Parmesan cheese
- 1 egg
- 2 cloves garlic, minced
- 1 teaspoon dried oregano
- 1 teaspoon dried basil
- Salt and pepper to taste
- 2 large zucchinis, spiralized into noodles
- 2 tablespoons olive oil
- 1 cup marinara sauce

- Fresh basil leaves, for garnish

Preparation:

In a mixing bowl, combine ground turkey, breadcrumbs, grated Parmesan cheese, minced garlic, dried oregano, dried basil, salt, and pepper. Mix well until all ingredients are evenly incorporated. Shape the mixture into meatballs of desired size. In a skillet, heat olive oil over medium heat and cook the meatballs until browned and cooked through. Remove the meatballs from the skillet and set aside. In the same skillet, add the spiralized zucchini noodles and sauté for a few minutes until they are tender but still slightly crunchy. Pour the marinara sauce over the zucchini noodles and heat until warmed through. Serve the zucchini noodles topped with the turkey meatballs and garnish with fresh basil leaves.

Spicy Turkey Meatballs with Garlic Zucchini Noodles:

Ingredients:

- 1 pound ground turkey
- 1/2 cup panko breadcrumbs
- 1/4 cup grated Pecorino Romano cheese
- 1 egg
- 2 cloves garlic, minced

- 1 teaspoon chili powder
- 1/2 teaspoon cayenne pepper
- Salt and pepper to taste
- 2 large zucchinis, spiralized into noodles
- 2 tablespoons olive oil
- 2 tablespoons butter
- Fresh parsley, for garnish

Preparation:

In a mixing bowl, combine ground turkey, panko breadcrumbs, grated Pecorino Romano cheese, minced garlic, chili powder, cayenne pepper, salt, and pepper. Mix well until all ingredients are evenly incorporated. Shape the mixture into meatballs and set aside. In a skillet, heat olive oil over medium heat and cook the meatballs until browned and cooked through. Remove the meatballs from the skillet and set aside. In the same skillet, add butter and sauté the spiralized zucchini noodles until they are tender. Serve the zucchini noodles topped with the spicy turkey meatballs and garnish with fresh parsley.

Asian-Inspired Turkey Meatballs with Sesame Zucchini Noodles:

Ingredients:

- 1 pound ground turkey
- 1/2 cup panko breadcrumbs

- 1/4 cup chopped green onions
- 2 cloves garlic, minced
- 1 teaspoon grated fresh ginger
- 2 tablespoons soy sauce
- 1 tablespoon hoisin sauce
- Salt and pepper to taste
- 2 large zucchinis, spiralized into noodles
- 2 tablespoons sesame oil
- 1 tablespoon toasted sesame seeds
- Fresh cilantro, for garnish

Preparation:

In a mixing bowl, combine ground turkey, panko breadcrumbs, chopped green onions, minced garlic, grated fresh ginger, soy sauce, hoisin sauce, salt, and pepper. Mix well until all ingredients are evenly incorporated. Shape the mixture into meatballs and set aside. In a skillet, heat sesame oil over medium heat and cook the meatballs until browned and cooked through. Remove the meatballs from the skillet and set aside. In the same skillet, add the spiralized zucchini noodles and sauté until they are tender. Serve the zucchini noodles topped with the Asian-inspired turkey meatballs and garnish with toasted sesame seeds and fresh cilantro.

**Italian Turkey Meatballs with Tomato-Basil
Zucchini Noodles:**

Ingredients:

- 1 pound ground turkey
- 1/2 cup breadcrumbs
- 1/4 cup grated Parmesan cheese
- 1 egg
- 2 cloves garlic, minced
- 1 teaspoon dried oregano
- 1 teaspoon dried basil
- Salt and pepper to taste
- 2 large zucchinis, spiralized into noodles
- 2 tablespoons olive oil
- 1 cup cherry tomatoes, halved
- Fresh basil leaves, for garnish

Preparation:

In a mixing bowl, combine ground turkey, breadcrumbs, grated Parmesan cheese, minced garlic, dried oregano, dried basil, salt, and pepper. Mix well until all ingredients are evenly incorporated. Shape the mixture into meatballs and set aside. In a skillet, heat olive oil over medium heat and cook the meatballs until browned and cooked through. Remove the meatballs from the skillet and set aside. In the same skillet, add the spiralized zucchini noodles and halved cherry tomatoes. Sauté until the zucchini noodles are tender and the cherry tomatoes are slightly softened. Serve the zucchini noodles topped with the Italian turkey meatballs and garnish with fresh basil leaves.

Greek-Inspired Turkey Meatballs with Tzatziki Zucchini Noodles:

Ingredients:

- 1 pound ground turkey
- 1/2 cup breadcrumbs
- 1/4 cup crumbled feta cheese
- 1 egg
- 2 cloves garlic, minced
- 1 teaspoon dried oregano
- 1 teaspoon dried dill
- Salt and pepper to taste
- 2 large zucchinis, spiralized into noodles
- 2 tablespoons olive oil
- 1/2 cup Greek yogurt
- 1/4 cup grated cucumber
- 1 tablespoon lemon juice
- Fresh dill, for garnish

Preparation:

In a mixing bowl, combine ground turkey, breadcrumbs, crumbled feta cheese, minced garlic, dried oregano, dried dill, salt, and pepper. Mix well until all ingredients are evenly incorporated. Shape the mixture into meatballs and set aside. In a skillet, heat olive oil over medium heat and cook the meatballs until browned and cooked through. Remove the meatballs from the skillet and set aside. In a small bowl, mix Greek yogurt, grated cucumber, and lemon juice to make the tzatziki sauce. In the same skillet, add the spiralized zucchini noodles and sauté until they are tender. Serve the zucchini noodles topped with the Greek-inspired turkey meatballs and drizzle with the tzatziki sauce. Garnish with fresh dill.

These 100% unique and flavorful Turkey Meatballs with Zucchini Noodles recipes are the perfect combination of protein and veggies, providing a delicious and satisfying dinner option. Each dish features a distinct blend of herbs, spices, and sauces that elevate the turkey meatballs and complement the zucchini noodles, offering a burst of flavor and nutrition in every bite. So, indulge in these healthy and hearty dishes, and treat yourself to a delightful dinner that's both wholesome and delicious!

Lentil and Vegetable Curry

Spicy Red Lentil and Vegetable Curry:

Ingredients:

- 1 cup red lentils
- 1 tablespoon vegetable oil

- 1 onion, chopped
- 3 cloves garlic, minced
- 1 tablespoon grated ginger
- 1 teaspoon ground cumin
- 1 teaspoon ground coriander
- 1 teaspoon turmeric
- 1/2 teaspoon cayenne pepper (optional for added spice)
- 2 cups mixed vegetables (such as carrots, bell peppers, and peas)
- 1 can (14 ounces) diced tomatoes
- 1 can (13.5 ounces) coconut milk
- Salt and pepper to taste
- Fresh cilantro, for garnish
- Cooked rice or naan bread, for serving

Preparation:

Rinse the red lentils under cold water and set aside. In a large pot, heat the vegetable oil over medium heat. Add the chopped onion and sauté until translucent. Add the minced garlic, grated ginger, ground cumin, ground coriander, turmeric, and cayenne pepper (if using), and cook for another minute until fragrant. Add the mixed vegetables, diced tomatoes (with their juice), coconut milk, and rinsed red lentils to the pot. Stir well to combine. Bring the mixture to a boil, then reduce the heat and simmer for about 20-25 minutes, or until the lentils and vegetables are tender. Season with salt and pepper to taste. Serve the spicy red lentil and vegetable curry over cooked rice or with naan bread. Garnish with fresh cilantro.

Coconut Curry Lentil Soup with Roasted Vegetables:

Ingredients:

- 1 cup green lentils
- 1 tablespoon vegetable oil
- 1 onion, chopped
- 3 cloves garlic, minced
- 1 tablespoon grated ginger
- 2 tablespoons curry powder
- 1 teaspoon ground cumin
- 1 can (13.5 ounces) coconut milk
- 4 cups vegetable broth
- 2 cups roasted vegetables (such as cauliflower, carrots, and bell peppers)
- Salt and pepper to taste
- Fresh cilantro, for garnish

Preparation:

Rinse the green lentils under cold water and set aside. In a large pot, heat the vegetable oil over medium heat. Add the chopped onion and sauté until translucent. Add the minced garlic, grated ginger, curry powder, and ground cumin, and cook for another minute until fragrant. Add the rinsed green lentils, coconut milk, and vegetable broth to the pot. Stir well to combine. Bring the mixture to a boil, then reduce the heat and simmer for about 30-35 minutes, or until the lentils are tender. Add the roasted vegetables to the soup and cook for another 5 minutes to heat through. Season with salt and pepper to taste. Serve the coconut curry lentil soup with roasted vegetables garnished with fresh cilantro.

Moroccan Lentil and Vegetable Tagine:

Ingredients:

- 1 cup brown lentils
- 1 tablespoon olive oil
- 1 onion, chopped
- 3 cloves garlic, minced
- 1 tablespoon ras el hanout spice blend
- 1 teaspoon ground cumin
- 1 teaspoon ground coriander
- 1 teaspoon ground cinnamon
- 2 cups chopped mixed vegetables (such as eggplant, zucchini, and bell peppers)
- 1 can (14 ounces) diced tomatoes
- 2 cups vegetable broth
- Salt and pepper to taste
- Fresh parsley, for garnish
- Cooked couscous, for serving

Preparation:

Rinse the brown lentils under cold water and set aside. In a large pot, heat the olive oil over medium heat. Add the chopped onion and sauté until translucent. Add the minced garlic, ras el hanout spice blend, ground cumin, ground coriander, and ground cinnamon, and cook for another minute until fragrant. Add the chopped mixed vegetables, diced tomatoes (with their juice), rinsed brown lentils, and vegetable broth to the pot. Stir well to combine. Bring the mixture to a boil, then reduce the heat and simmer for about 35-40 minutes, or until the lentils and vegetables are tender. Season with salt and pepper to taste. Serve the Moroccan lentil and vegetable tagine over cooked couscous and garnish with fresh parsley.

Thai Red Curry Lentil Stir-Fry:

Ingredients:

- 1 cup red lentils
- 1 tablespoon vegetable oil
- 1 onion, sliced
- 1 red bell pepper, sliced
- 1 cup sliced mushrooms
- 1 cup snap peas
- 2 tablespoons Thai red curry paste
- 1 can (13.5 ounces) coconut milk
- 1 tablespoon soy sauce

- 1 tablespoon lime juice
- Fresh cilantro and lime wedges, for garnish
- Cooked rice or noodles, for serving

Preparation:

Rinse the red lentils under cold water and set aside. In a large skillet or wok, heat the vegetable oil over medium heat. Add the sliced onion, red bell pepper, mushrooms, and snap peas to the skillet and stir-fry for about 5-6 minutes, or until the vegetables are tender-crisp. Add the Thai red curry paste to the skillet and stir-fry for another minute to coat the vegetables. Add the rinsed red lentils, coconut milk, soy sauce, and lime juice to the skillet. Stir well to combine. Simmer the mixture for about 10-15 minutes, or until the lentils are cooked through and the flavors have melded together. Serve the Thai red curry lentil stir-fry over cooked rice or noodles. Garnish with fresh cilantro and lime wedges.

Indian Dal with Mixed Vegetables:

Ingredients:

- 1 cup yellow split peas (dal)
- 1 tablespoon ghee or vegetable oil
- 1 onion, chopped
- 3 cloves garlic, minced
- 1 tablespoon grated ginger

- 1 teaspoon ground cumin
- 1 teaspoon ground coriander
- 1/2 teaspoon turmeric
- 2 cups mixed vegetables (such as carrots, potatoes, and cauliflower)
- 4 cups vegetable broth
- Salt and pepper to taste
- Fresh cilantro, for garnish
- Cooked rice or naan bread, for serving

Preparation:

Rinse the yellow split peas under cold water and set aside. In a large pot, heat the ghee or vegetable oil over medium heat. Add the chopped onion and sauté until translucent. Add the minced garlic, grated ginger, ground cumin, ground coriander, and turmeric, and cook for another minute until fragrant. Add the mixed vegetables, rinsed yellow split peas, and vegetable broth to the pot. Stir well to combine. Bring the mixture to a boil, then reduce the heat and simmer for about 25-30 minutes, or until the split peas and vegetables are tender. Season with salt and pepper to taste. Serve the Indian dal with mixed vegetables over cooked rice or with naan bread. Garnish with fresh cilantro.

These 100% unique and delectable Lentil and Vegetable Curry recipes showcase the versatility and nutritious goodness of lentils combined with a variety of colorful vegetables and aromatic spices. Each dish offers a burst of flavor and a healthy dose of plant-based protein, making them perfect additions to your culinary repertoire. So, savor the taste of these hearty and satisfying curries, and embrace the wonderful world of lentils and veggies for a wholesome and nourishing dining experience!

Chapter 5

Delicious Snacks and Appetizers

Welcome to the world of Delicious Snacks and Appetizers, where taste meets creativity and convenience. In this collection of delectable recipes, we'll explore a delightful assortment of appetizers and snacks that are not only incredibly flavorful but also easy to prepare. Whether you're hosting a party, looking for quick bites to satisfy your cravings, or seeking wholesome options to enjoy with loved ones, these recipes have got you covered.

Snacking has never been this exciting, as we venture into a journey of flavors and textures that will tantalize your taste buds. From savory to sweet, from crunchy to creamy, our hand-picked recipes offer a wide variety of options to suit every palate and occasion. Whether you're a seasoned chef or a kitchen enthusiast, you'll find these recipes approachable and enjoyable to recreate.

Indulge in the rich flavors of Mediterranean-inspired hummus rolls, savor the crunchy goodness of spiced roasted chickpeas, and treat yourself to refreshing cucumber and hummus combinations. As we explore these delectable appetizers and snacks, you'll discover that healthy eating doesn't mean compromising on taste. Each recipe is carefully crafted to provide a balance of nutrients and flavors, making them not only delicious but also nourishing.

So, get ready to embark on a culinary adventure filled with mouthwatering creations that will impress your guests, delight your family, and become your go-to treats. Whether you're seeking a light and refreshing bite or a satisfying and wholesome snack, these recipes are sure to become your new favorites. Let's dive in and discover the joy of creating these scrumptious snacks and appetizers in your very own kitchen!

Avocado and Tomato Bruschetta:

Ingredients:

- 1 baguette, sliced
- 2 ripe avocados, mashed
- 1 cup cherry tomatoes, diced
- 1/4 cup red onion, finely chopped
- 2 tablespoons fresh basil, chopped
- 1 tablespoon balsamic vinegar
- 2 tablespoons olive oil
- Salt and pepper to taste

Preparation:

Preheat the oven to 375°F (190°C). Arrange the baguette slices on a baking sheet and lightly brush them with olive oil. Bake for 5-7 minutes or until they become slightly crispy. In a mixing bowl, combine the mashed avocados, diced tomatoes, red onion, chopped basil, balsamic vinegar, and olive oil. Season with salt and pepper. Top each baguette slice with the avocado-tomato mixture. Serve the avocado and tomato bruschetta as a delightful appetizer.

Baked Sweet Potato Fries:

Ingredients:

- 2 large sweet potatoes, cut into strips
- 2 tablespoons olive oil
- 1 teaspoon paprika
- 1 teaspoon garlic powder
- 1/2 teaspoon salt
- 1/4 teaspoon black pepper

Preparation:

Preheat the oven to 425°F (220°C). In a large mixing bowl, toss the sweet potato strips with olive oil, paprika, garlic powder, salt, and black pepper until they are well coated. Arrange the sweet potato strips on a baking sheet lined with parchment paper. Bake for 25-30 minutes or until the fries are crispy and golden brown. Serve the baked sweet potato fries with your favorite dipping sauce.

Spicy Chickpea Snack Mix:

Ingredients:

- 1 can (15 ounces) chickpeas, drained and rinsed
- 1 tablespoon olive oil
- 1 teaspoon ground cumin
- 1/2 teaspoon chili powder
- 1/2 teaspoon garlic powder
- 1/4 teaspoon cayenne pepper (adjust to taste)
- Salt to taste
- 1/4 cup dried cranberries
- 1/4 cup roasted almonds

Preparation:

Preheat the oven to 400°F (200°C). In a bowl, toss the chickpeas with olive oil, ground cumin, chili powder, garlic powder, cayenne pepper, and salt until they are well coated. Spread the seasoned chickpeas on a baking sheet lined with parchment paper. Bake for 20-25 minutes or until they become crispy. Remove the chickpeas from the oven and let them cool slightly. Mix in the dried cranberries and roasted almonds. Enjoy the spicy chickpea snack mix as a satisfying and nutritious snack.

Stuffed Mini Bell Peppers:

Ingredients:

- 10-12 mini bell peppers, halved and seeds removed
- 1 cup cooked quinoa
- 1/2 cup black beans, drained and rinsed
- 1/2 cup corn kernels
- 1/4 cup red onion, finely chopped
- 1/4 cup cherry tomatoes, diced
- 1/4 cup fresh cilantro, chopped
- 1 tablespoon lime juice
- 1 teaspoon ground cumin
- Salt and pepper to taste

Preparation:

In a large mixing bowl, combine the cooked quinoa, black beans, corn kernels, red onion, cherry tomatoes, cilantro, lime juice, ground cumin, salt, and pepper. Mix well until all ingredients are combined. Stuff each mini bell pepper half with the quinoa mixture. Arrange the stuffed peppers on a serving platter. Serve the stuffed mini bell peppers as a colorful and delightful appetizer.

Zucchini Fritters with Yogurt Sauce:

Ingredients:

- 2 medium zucchinis, grated and squeezed to remove excess moisture
- 1/4 cup grated Parmesan cheese
- 1/4 cup breadcrumbs
- 1 egg, lightly beaten
- 2 tablespoons fresh parsley, chopped
- 1/2 teaspoon garlic powder
- Salt and pepper to taste
- 2 tablespoons olive oil
- 1/2 cup Greek yogurt
- 1 tablespoon lemon juice
- 1 tablespoon fresh dill, chopped

Preparation:

In a large mixing bowl, combine the grated zucchinis, grated Parmesan cheese, breadcrumbs, beaten egg, chopped parsley, garlic powder, salt, and pepper. Mix well until all ingredients are evenly incorporated. Heat olive oil in a skillet over medium heat. Drop spoonfuls of the zucchini mixture into the skillet and flatten them slightly with a spatula to form fritters. Cook for 2-3 minutes on each side or until they become golden brown and crispy. In a small bowl, mix the Greek yogurt, lemon juice, and chopped dill to make the yogurt sauce. Serve the zucchini fritters with the refreshing yogurt sauce on the side.

These 100% unique and mouthwatering Snacks and Appetizers recipes offer a delightful array of flavors and textures to satisfy your cravings. From the creamy goodness of avocado and tomato bruschetta to the crunchy and spiced chickpea snack mix, each recipe brings a burst of taste and nutrition to your table. Whether you're entertaining guests or simply enjoying a light snack, these recipes will surely impress and leave everyone craving for more. So, get ready to indulge in these scrumptious treats and add a touch of excitement to your snack time!

Fresh Tomato Bruschetta

Classic Tomato and Basil Bruschetta:

Ingredients:

- 1 baguette, sliced
- 4-5 ripe tomatoes, diced
- 3 cloves garlic, minced
- 1/4 cup fresh basil leaves, chopped
- 2 tablespoons balsamic vinegar
- 2 tablespoons extra-virgin olive oil
- Salt and pepper to taste

Preparation:

Preheat the oven to 375°F (190°C). Arrange the baguette slices on a baking sheet and lightly brush them with olive oil. Bake for 5-7 minutes or until they become slightly crispy. In a mixing bowl, combine the diced tomatoes, minced garlic, chopped basil, balsamic vinegar, and olive oil. Season with salt and pepper. Top each baguette slice with the tomato-basil mixture. Serve the classic tomato and basil bruschetta as a refreshing appetizer.

Roasted Tomato and Mozzarella Bruschetta:

Ingredients:

- 1 baguette, sliced
- 2 cups cherry tomatoes
- 3 cloves garlic, minced
- 2 tablespoons balsamic vinegar
- 2 tablespoons extra-virgin olive oil
- 1 cup fresh mozzarella, diced
- 1/4 cup fresh basil leaves, chopped
- Salt and pepper to taste

Preparation:

Preheat the oven to 400°F (200°C). Place the cherry tomatoes on a baking sheet and drizzle with olive oil. Roast for 15-20 minutes or until the tomatoes start to burst and caramelize. In a mixing bowl, combine the roasted tomatoes, minced garlic, balsamic vinegar, and olive oil. Season with salt and pepper. Arrange the baguette slices on a serving platter and top each slice with diced mozzarella. Spoon the roasted tomato mixture over the mozzarella. Garnish with chopped basil. Serve the roasted tomato and mozzarella bruschetta for a delightful blend of flavors.

Avocado and Tomato Bruschetta with Feta:

Ingredients:

- 1 baguette, sliced
- 2 ripe avocados, mashed
- 1 cup cherry tomatoes, diced
- 1/4 cup red onion, finely chopped
- 2 tablespoons fresh cilantro, chopped
- 1 tablespoon lime juice
- 1/2 cup crumbled feta cheese
- Salt and pepper to taste

Preparation:

Preheat the oven to 375°F (190°C). Arrange the baguette slices on a baking sheet and lightly brush them with olive oil. Bake for 5-7 minutes or until they become slightly crispy. In a mixing bowl, combine the mashed avocados, diced tomatoes, red onion, chopped cilantro, and lime juice. Season with salt and pepper. Top each baguette slice with the avocado-tomato mixture. Sprinkle crumbled feta cheese over the top. Serve the avocado and tomato bruschetta with feta for a creamy and tangy twist.

Sun-Dried Tomato and Olive Tapenade Bruschetta:

Ingredients:

- 1 baguette, sliced
- 1/2 cup sun-dried tomatoes, rehydrated and chopped
- 1/4 cup black olives, pitted and chopped
- 2 tablespoons capers, drained
- 2 cloves garlic, minced
- 2 tablespoons fresh parsley, chopped
- 1 tablespoon lemon juice
- 2 tablespoons extra-virgin olive oil
- Salt and pepper to taste

Preparation:

Preheat the oven to 375°F (190°C). Arrange the baguette slices on a baking sheet and lightly brush them with olive oil. Bake for 5-7 minutes or until they become slightly crispy. In a food processor, combine the rehydrated sun-dried tomatoes, black olives, capers, minced garlic, chopped parsley, lemon juice, and olive oil. Pulse until the mixture forms a chunky tapenade. Season with salt and pepper. Spread the tapenade on each baguette slice. Serve the sun-dried tomato and olive tapenade bruschetta for a flavorful and savory delight.

Goat Cheese and Tomato Bruschetta with Balsamic Glaze:

Ingredients:

- 1 baguette, sliced
- 2 cups cherry tomatoes, halved
- 3 tablespoons balsamic vinegar
- 1 tablespoon honey
- 4 ounces goat cheese
- 2 tablespoons fresh basil, chopped
- Salt and pepper to taste

Preparation:

Preheat the oven to 375°F (190°C). Arrange the baguette slices on a baking sheet and lightly brush them with olive oil. Bake for 5-7 minutes or until they become slightly crispy. In a small saucepan, combine the balsamic vinegar and honey. Bring to a simmer over medium heat and cook for 3-4 minutes, or until the mixture thickens and reduces to a glaze. In a mixing bowl, toss the cherry tomatoes with the balsamic glaze. Spread goat cheese on each baguette slice. Top with the balsamic-coated tomatoes. Garnish with chopped basil. Serve the goat cheese and tomato bruschetta with balsamic glaze for a sweet and tangy flavor combination.

These 100% unique and delectable Fresh Tomato Bruschetta recipes offer a burst of vibrant flavors and a delightful array of textures. From the classic tomato and basil bruschetta to the sun-dried tomato and olive tapenade, each recipe brings a unique twist to this Italian-inspired appetizer. So, whether you're hosting a gathering or simply looking for a quick and satisfying snack, these bruschetta recipes are sure to impress and delight your taste buds. Enjoy the fresh goodness of tomatoes paired with various mouthwatering ingredients for a delightful culinary experience!

Cucumber and Hummus Roll-Ups

Classic Cucumber and Hummus Roll-Ups:

Ingredients:

- 1 large cucumber
- 1 cup hummus
- 1/4 cup shredded carrots
- 1/4 cup alfalfa sprouts
- Salt and pepper to taste

Preparation:

 Using a vegetable peeler, thinly slice the cucumber lengthwise into long strips. Lay the cucumber slices flat on a clean surface. Spread a generous amount of hummus on each cucumber slice. Sprinkle shredded carrots and alfalfa sprouts evenly over the hummus. Season with salt and pepper to taste. Gently roll up each cucumber slice to form a tight roll. Secure the roll-ups with toothpicks if needed. Serve the classic cucumber and hummus roll-ups as a refreshing and nutritious snack.

Mediterranean Cucumber and Hummus Roll-Ups:

Ingredients:

- 1 large cucumber
- 1 cup roasted red pepper hummus
- 1/4 cup Kalamata olives, pitted and chopped
- 1/4 cup crumbled feta cheese
- 2 tablespoons fresh parsley, chopped
- 1 tablespoon lemon juice
- Salt and pepper to taste

Preparation:

Thinly slice the cucumber lengthwise into long strips using a vegetable peeler. Lay the cucumber slices flat on a clean surface. Spread roasted red pepper hummus on each cucumber slice. Sprinkle chopped Kalamata olives, crumbled feta cheese, and chopped parsley over the hummus. Drizzle lemon juice over the toppings. Season with salt and pepper to taste. Carefully roll up each cucumber slice to form a delicious Mediterranean-inspired roll-up. Serve the cucumber and hummus roll-ups for a burst of Mediterranean flavors.

Thai-Inspired Cucumber and Hummus Roll-Ups:

Ingredients:

- 1 large cucumber
- 1 cup Thai curry hummus
- 1/4 cup shredded purple cabbage
- 1/4 cup julienned carrots
- 2 tablespoons chopped fresh cilantro
- 1 tablespoon lime juice
- Crushed peanuts (optional)
- Salt and pepper to taste

Preparation:

Using a vegetable peeler, thinly slice the cucumber lengthwise into long strips. Lay the cucumber slices flat on a clean surface. Spread Thai curry hummus on each cucumber slice. Sprinkle shredded purple cabbage, julienned carrots, and chopped cilantro over the hummus. Drizzle lime juice over the toppings. Add crushed peanuts for an extra crunch if desired. Season with salt and pepper to taste. Roll up each cucumber slice to create Thai-inspired roll-ups bursting with vibrant flavors.

Greek Cucumber and Hummus Roll-Ups:

Ingredients:

- 1 large cucumber
- 1 cup tzatziki hummus
- 1/4 cup cherry tomatoes, halved
- 1/4 cup diced cucumber
- 2 tablespoons sliced black olives
- 2 tablespoons crumbled feta cheese
- 1 tablespoon fresh dill, chopped
- Salt and pepper to taste

Preparation:

Thinly slice the cucumber lengthwise into long strips using a vegetable peeler. Lay the cucumber slices flat on a clean surface. Spread tzatziki hummus on each cucumber slice. Arrange halved cherry tomatoes, diced cucumber, sliced black olives, and crumbled feta cheese over the hummus. Sprinkle fresh dill on top. Season with salt and pepper to taste. Roll up each cucumber slice to create Greek-inspired roll-ups with a burst of Mediterranean flavors.

Avocado and Cucumber Hummus Roll-Ups:

Ingredients:

- 1 large cucumber
- 1 ripe avocado, mashed
- 1 cup plain hummus
- 1/4 cup baby spinach leaves
- 1/4 cup thinly sliced red bell pepper
- 2 tablespoons chopped fresh chives
- 1 tablespoon lime juice
- Salt and pepper to taste

Preparation:

Using a vegetable peeler, thinly slice the cucumber lengthwise into long strips. Lay the cucumber slices flat on a clean surface. In a small bowl, mix the mashed avocado and lime juice until well combined. Spread a layer of plain hummus on each cucumber slice. Top with the avocado mixture, baby spinach leaves, sliced red bell pepper, and chopped chives. Season with salt and pepper to taste. Roll up each cucumber slice to create avocado and cucumber hummus roll-ups with a creamy and nutritious filling.

These 100% unique Cucumber and Hummus Roll-Ups recipes offer a delightful combination of fresh cucumber and creamy hummus with a variety of delicious toppings and flavors. From classic combinations to international inspirations, each roll-up brings a burst of taste and nutrition to your table. Whether you're hosting a party or enjoying a light and satisfying snack, these roll-ups are sure to impress and leave everyone wanting more. So, roll up these delectable treats and savor the goodness of cucumber and hummus in every bite!

Spiced Roasted Chickpeas

Classic Spiced Roasted Chickpeas:

Ingredients:

- 1 can (15 ounces) chickpeas, drained and rinsed
- 1 tablespoon olive oil
- 1 teaspoon ground cumin
- 1/2 teaspoon chili powder
- 1/2 teaspoon paprika
- 1/4 teaspoon garlic powder
- Salt and pepper to taste

Preparation:

Preheat the oven to 400°F (200°C). In a bowl, toss the chickpeas with olive oil, ground cumin, chili powder, paprika, garlic powder, salt, and pepper until well coated. Spread the chickpeas in a single layer on a baking sheet lined with parchment paper. Roast in the oven for 20-25 minutes or until the chickpeas become crispy and golden brown. Shake the baking sheet halfway through to ensure even roasting. Remove from the oven and let them cool slightly before serving. Enjoy the classic spiced roasted chickpeas as a flavorful and crunchy snack!

Smoky BBQ Roasted Chickpeas:

Ingredients:

- 1 can (15 ounces) chickpeas, drained and rinsed
- 1 tablespoon olive oil
- 1 teaspoon smoked paprika
- 1/2 teaspoon onion powder
- 1/2 teaspoon ground cumin
- 1/4 teaspoon cayenne pepper (optional, for added heat)
- 1/4 teaspoon sea salt

Preparation:

Preheat the oven to 400°F (200°C). In a bowl, toss the chickpeas with olive oil, smoked paprika, onion powder, ground cumin, cayenne pepper (if using), and sea salt until evenly coated. Spread the chickpeas in a single layer on a baking sheet lined with parchment paper. Roast in the oven for 20-25 minutes or until the chickpeas are crispy and slightly charred. Shake the baking sheet halfway through to ensure even roasting. Let the smoky BBQ roasted chickpeas cool for a few minutes before serving. Enjoy the bold and smoky flavors of this savory snack!

Sweet and Spicy Roasted Chickpeas:

Ingredients:

- 1 can (15 ounces) chickpeas, drained and rinsed
- 1 tablespoon olive oil
- 1 tablespoon maple syrup
- 1/2 teaspoon ground cinnamon
- 1/4 teaspoon cayenne pepper
- 1/4 teaspoon sea salt

Preparation:

Preheat the oven to 375°F (190°C). In a bowl, toss the chickpeas with olive oil, maple syrup, ground cinnamon, cayenne pepper, and sea salt until well coated. Spread the chickpeas in a single layer on a baking sheet lined with parchment paper. Roast in the oven for 25-30 minutes or until the chickpeas are crispy and caramelized. Stir the chickpeas occasionally during roasting to prevent sticking. Allow the sweet and spicy roasted chickpeas to cool before serving. Enjoy the perfect balance of sweet and heat in this delightful snack!

Herbed Garlic Roasted Chickpeas:

Ingredients:

- 1 can (15 ounces) chickpeas, drained and rinsed
- 2 tablespoons olive oil
- 2 cloves garlic, minced
- 1 teaspoon dried thyme
- 1 teaspoon dried rosemary
- 1/2 teaspoon dried oregano
- 1/4 teaspoon sea salt
- Freshly ground black pepper to taste

Preparation:

Preheat the oven to 375°F (190°C). In a bowl, toss the chickpeas with olive oil, minced garlic, dried thyme, dried rosemary, dried oregano, sea salt, and black pepper until evenly coated. Spread the chickpeas in a single layer on a baking sheet lined with parchment paper. Roast in the oven for 20-25 minutes or until the chickpeas are crispy and infused with herb and garlic flavors. Stir the chickpeas occasionally during roasting to ensure even cooking. Let the herbed garlic roasted chickpeas cool down before serving. Enjoy the aromatic and savory goodness of this herby snack!

Curry-Spiced Roasted Chickpeas:

Ingredients:

- 1 can (15 ounces) chickpeas, drained and rinsed
- 1 tablespoon olive oil
- 1 tablespoon curry powder
- 1/2 teaspoon ground turmeric
- 1/4 teaspoon ground cumin
- 1/4 teaspoon ground coriander
- 1/4 teaspoon sea salt

Preparation:

Preheat the oven to 375°F (190°C). In a bowl, toss the chickpeas with olive oil, curry powder, ground turmeric, ground cumin, ground coriander, and sea salt until well coated. Spread the chickpeas in a single layer on a baking sheet lined with parchment paper. Roast in the oven for 25-30 minutes or until the chickpeas are crispy and infused with aromatic curry flavors. Stir the chickpeas occasionally during roasting to prevent burning. Let the curry-spiced roasted chickpeas cool before serving. Enjoy the delightful blend of spices in this exotic and flavorful snack!

These 100% unique Spiced Roasted Chickpeas recipes offer a diverse array of flavors, from classic spices to adventurous blends, all combined with the irresistible crunch of roasted chickpeas. These versatile snacks can be enjoyed on their own, sprinkled over salads, or added to your favorite dishes for an extra kick. Whether you prefer sweet, smoky, or savory flavors, these recipes have something to satisfy every taste bud. So, get ready to indulge in the delightful goodness of these spiced roasted chickpeas, packed with protein and bold flavors to keep you coming back for more!

Chapter 6

Sweet Treats with Low-GI Goodness

Indulge your sweet tooth guilt-free with "Sweet Treats with Low-GI Goodness," a delightful collection of mouthwatering desserts that are not only delicious but also low on the glycemic index (GI). In this book, we'll explore a world of sweetness that won't cause sharp spikes in blood sugar levels, making it a perfect choice for those seeking healthier options without compromising on taste.

The glycemic index is a valuable tool in managing blood sugar levels, and our recipes are thoughtfully crafted to feature ingredients with low GI values. From fruity delights to decadent chocolate creations, each dessert is carefully designed to keep your blood sugar in check while satisfying your cravings for sweetness.

In this sweet journey, you'll discover the wonders of using natural sweeteners and nutrient-rich ingredients that not only contribute to the delightful flavors but also provide a nourishing boost. From the subtle sweetness of fresh fruits to the richness of wholesome nuts and seeds, our recipes celebrate the beauty of whole foods in creating delectable treats.

Whether you're managing diabetes, trying to make healthier dessert choices, or simply looking for innovative recipes to enjoy, "Sweet Treats with Low-GI Goodness" offers a range of options to suit every occasion and dietary preference. From simple and quick-to-make desserts to show-stopping delights, these recipes are suitable for all skill levels and will leave a lasting impression on your taste buds.

So, let's embark on a sweet adventure that celebrates the goodness of low-GI treats without compromising on the joy of indulgence. Get ready to savor every mouthful of these delightful creations that nourish your body and satisfy your soul with every sweet bite!

Dark Chocolate Avocado Truffles

Classic Dark Chocolate Avocado Truffles:

Ingredients:

- 1 ripe avocado
- 1 cup dark chocolate chips
- 2 tablespoons unsweetened cocoa powder
- 1 teaspoon vanilla extract
- Pinch of salt
- Optional toppings: chopped nuts, shredded coconut, or cocoa powder for rolling

Preparation:

In a microwave-safe bowl, melt the dark chocolate chips in 30-second intervals, stirring in between, until smooth and creamy.

In a separate bowl, mash the ripe avocado until no lumps remain.

Add the melted chocolate, unsweetened cocoa powder, vanilla extract, and a pinch of salt to the mashed avocado. Mix until well combined and a smooth, thick mixture forms.

Cover the bowl and refrigerate the mixture for at least 1 hour to firm up.

Once the mixture is firm, use a spoon or a small cookie scoop to portion out the truffles.

Roll each portion into a ball and coat them with your desired toppings, such as chopped nuts, shredded coconut, or cocoa powder.

Place the coated truffles on a parchment-lined tray and refrigerate for an additional 15-30 minutes to set.

Serve the classic dark chocolate avocado truffles chilled, and enjoy the creamy, decadent goodness!

Minty Dark Chocolate Avocado Truffles:

Ingredients:

- 1 ripe avocado
- 1 cup dark chocolate chips
- 2 tablespoons unsweetened cocoa powder
- 1/2 teaspoon peppermint extract
- Pinch of salt
- Green food coloring (optional)
- Optional toppings: crushed peppermint candy or melted white chocolate drizzle

Preparation:

Follow the same steps for melting the dark chocolate chips as in the Classic Dark Chocolate Avocado Truffles recipe.

In a separate bowl, mash the ripe avocado until smooth.

Add the melted chocolate, unsweetened cocoa powder, peppermint extract, and a pinch of salt to the mashed avocado. Mix until well combined. Add green food coloring, if desired, for a vibrant green hue.

Cover the bowl and refrigerate the mixture for at least 1 hour to firm up.

Once the mixture is firm, use a spoon or cookie scoop to portion out the truffles.

Roll each portion into a ball and coat them with crushed peppermint candy or drizzle melted white chocolate on top for a festive touch.

Place the minty dark chocolate avocado truffles on a parchment-lined tray and refrigerate for an additional 15-30 minutes to set.

Serve these refreshing and minty truffles chilled, and relish the delightful combination of chocolate and mint flavors!

Orange and Almond Dark Chocolate Avocado Truffles:

Ingredients:

- 1 ripe avocado
- 1 cup dark chocolate chips
- 2 tablespoons unsweetened cocoa powder
- 1 teaspoon orange zest
- 1/2 teaspoon almond extract
- Pinch of salt
- Optional toppings: finely chopped almonds or orange zest

Preparation:

Melt the dark chocolate chips following the same method as in the previous recipes.

Mash the ripe avocado until smooth in a separate bowl.

Add the melted chocolate, unsweetened cocoa powder, orange zest, almond extract, and a pinch of salt to the mashed avocado. Mix until thoroughly combined.

Cover the bowl and refrigerate the mixture for at least 1 hour to firm up.

Once the mixture is firm, scoop out portions of the truffle mixture and shape them into balls.

Roll the truffles in finely chopped almonds or orange zest for added texture and flavor.

Place the orange and almond dark chocolate avocado truffles on a parchment-lined tray and refrigerate for an additional 15-30 minutes to set.

Serve these delightful truffles chilled, and experience the heavenly fusion of dark chocolate, orange, and almond!

Coconut Dark Chocolate Avocado Truffles:

Ingredients:

- 1 ripe avocado
- 1 cup dark chocolate chips
- 2 tablespoons unsweetened cocoa powder
- 1 teaspoon coconut extract

- Pinch of salt
- Shredded coconut (sweetened or unsweetened) for coating

Preparation:

Melt the dark chocolate chips as mentioned in the previous recipes.

In a separate bowl, mash the ripe avocado until creamy and free of lumps.

Add the melted chocolate, unsweetened cocoa powder, coconut extract, and a pinch of salt to the mashed avocado. Mix thoroughly until well combined.

Cover the bowl and refrigerate the mixture for at least 1 hour to firm up.

Once the mixture is firm, scoop out portions of the truffle mixture and shape them into balls.

Roll the truffles in shredded coconut, either sweetened or unsweetened, for a delightful coconut coating.

Place the coconut dark chocolate avocado truffles on a parchment-lined tray and refrigerate for an additional 15-30 minutes to set.

Serve these tropical-inspired truffles chilled, and enjoy the perfect harmony of coconut and dark chocolate!

Hazelnut Dark Chocolate Avocado Truffles:

Ingredients:

- 1 ripe avocado
- 1 cup dark chocolate chips
- 2 tablespoons unsweetened cocoa powder
- 1/2 cup finely ground toasted hazelnuts
- Pinch of salt
- Optional toppings: whole hazelnuts or cocoa powder for rolling

Preparation:

Melt the dark chocolate chips as described in the earlier recipes.

In a separate bowl, mash the ripe avocado until smooth and creamy.

Add the melted chocolate, unsweetened cocoa powder, finely ground toasted hazelnuts, and a pinch of salt to the mashed avocado. Mix until well combined.

Cover the bowl and refrigerate the mixture for at least 1 hour to firm up.

Once the mixture is firm, scoop out portions of the truffle mixture and shape them into balls.

Roll the truffles in whole hazelnuts or cocoa powder for a delightful and crunchy outer layer.

Place the hazelnut dark chocolate avocado truffles on a parchment-lined tray and refrigerate for an additional 15-30 minutes to set.

Serve these hazelnut-infused truffles chilled, and experience the delightful fusion of rich chocolate and nutty flavors!

Enjoy these delectable Dark Chocolate Avocado Truffles recipes that not only satisfy your sweet cravings but also offer a healthy twist with the goodness of avocado and low-GI ingredients. Whether it's a special occasion or a simple indulgence, these truffles are sure to impress your taste buds and leave you wanting more!

Coconut and Berry Chia Pudding

Classic Coconut and Mixed Berry Chia Pudding:

Ingredients:

- 1/4 cup chia seeds
- 1 cup coconut milk (full-fat or light, as per preference)
- 1 tablespoon maple syrup or honey (adjust sweetness to taste)
- 1/2 teaspoon vanilla extract
- 1/2 cup mixed berries (strawberries, blueberries, raspberries)

Preparation:

In a bowl, combine chia seeds, coconut milk, maple syrup (or honey), and vanilla extract. Mix well to ensure the chia seeds are evenly distributed.

Cover the bowl and refrigerate for at least 4 hours or overnight to allow the chia seeds to absorb the liquid and form a pudding-like consistency.

Before serving, give the mixture a good stir to break up any clumps and ensure a smooth texture.

Layer the chia pudding with fresh mixed berries in a serving glass or jar for a delightful and visually appealing treat.

Garnish with additional berries on top and serve the classic coconut and mixed berry chia pudding chilled. Enjoy the refreshing burst of berry goodness!

Tropical Coconut and Mango Chia Pudding:

Ingredients:

- 1/4 cup chia seeds
- 1 cup coconut milk (full-fat or light)
- 1 tablespoon agave nectar or sweetener of your choice
- 1/2 teaspoon coconut extract
- 1 ripe mango, diced

Preparation:

In a bowl, mix chia seeds, coconut milk, agave nectar (or sweetener), and coconut extract until well combined.

Cover the bowl and refrigerate for at least 4 hours or overnight, allowing the chia seeds to absorb the liquid and create a pudding-like consistency.

Before serving, stir the mixture to ensure a smooth texture.

Layer the chia pudding with diced ripe mango for a taste of the tropics in every spoonful.

Serve the tropical coconut and mango chia pudding chilled, and savor the exotic flavors of coconut and mango dancing on your taste buds!

Creamy Coconut and Raspberry Chia Pudding:

Ingredients:

- 1/4 cup chia seeds
- 1 cup coconut milk (full-fat or light)
- 1 tablespoon honey or sweetener of your choice
- 1/2 teaspoon almond extract
- 1/2 cup fresh raspberries

Preparation:

In a bowl, combine chia seeds, coconut milk, honey (or sweetener), and almond extract. Mix until well incorporated.

Cover the bowl and refrigerate for at least 4 hours or overnight, allowing the chia seeds to thicken and create a creamy pudding consistency.

Stir the mixture before serving to achieve a smooth texture.

Layer the chia pudding with fresh raspberries, creating a delightful contrast of creaminess and tangy sweetness.

Serve the creamy coconut and raspberry chia pudding chilled, and enjoy the luscious blend of flavors.

Decadent Chocolate Coconut and Strawberry Chia Pudding:

Ingredients:

- 1/4 cup chia seeds
- 1 cup coconut milk (full-fat or light)
- 2 tablespoons cocoa powder
- 2 tablespoons agave nectar or sweetener of your choice
- 1/2 teaspoon coconut extract
- 1/2 cup sliced strawberries

Preparation:

In a bowl, whisk chia seeds, coconut milk, cocoa powder, agave nectar (or sweetener), and coconut extract until well combined.

Cover the bowl and refrigerate for at least 4 hours or overnight, allowing the chia seeds to expand and create a velvety pudding texture.

Before serving, give the mixture a good stir to achieve a smooth consistency.

Layer the chocolate coconut chia pudding with sliced strawberries for a heavenly combination of flavors.

Serve the decadent chocolate coconut and strawberry chia pudding chilled, and experience a delightful interplay of chocolate and strawberry goodness.

Nutty Coconut and Blueberry Chia Pudding:

Ingredients:

- 1/4 cup chia seeds
- 1 cup coconut milk (full-fat or light)
- 1 tablespoon agave nectar or sweetener of your choice
- 1/2 teaspoon almond extract
- 1/4 cup fresh blueberries
- 2 tablespoons chopped almonds

Preparation:

In a bowl, mix chia seeds, coconut milk, agave nectar (or sweetener), and almond extract until well combined.

Cover the bowl and refrigerate for at least 4 hours or overnight, allowing the chia seeds to absorb the liquid and create a creamy pudding texture.

Stir the mixture before serving to achieve a smooth consistency.

Layer the coconut chia pudding with fresh blueberries and top with chopped almonds for a delightful crunch.

Serve the nutty coconut and blueberry chia pudding chilled, and relish the delightful contrast of flavors and textures.

These Coconut and Berry Chia Pudding recipes offer a harmonious blend of creamy coconut goodness and the natural sweetness of fresh berries, making them a delectable and healthy treat for any time of the day. Enjoy these nutrient-rich and flavorful puddings guilt-free, and indulge in the delightful benefits of chia seeds and the lusciousness of coconut and berries!

Almond Flour Blueberry Muffins

Classic Almond Flour Blueberry Muffins:

Ingredients:

- 2 cups almond flour
- 1/4 cup coconut flour
- 1/4 cup tapioca flour
- 1 teaspoon baking powder
- 1/4 teaspoon salt
- 3 large eggs
- 1/3 cup honey or maple syrup
- 1/3 cup coconut oil, melted
- 1 teaspoon vanilla extract
- 1 cup fresh blueberries

Preparation:

Preheat the oven to 350°F (175°C) and line a muffin tin with paper liners or grease each cup with coconut oil.

In a large mixing bowl, whisk together almond flour, coconut flour, tapioca flour, baking powder, and salt until well combined.

In a separate bowl, whisk the eggs, honey (or maple syrup), melted coconut oil, and vanilla extract until smooth.

Add the wet ingredients to the dry ingredients and mix until a thick batter forms.

Gently fold in the fresh blueberries, being careful not to overmix.

Divide the batter evenly among the muffin cups, filling each about 3/4 full.

Bake the muffins in the preheated oven for 20-25 minutes or until a toothpick inserted into the center comes out clean.

Allow the muffins to cool in the pan for a few minutes before transferring them to a wire rack to cool completely. Enjoy the classic almond flour blueberry muffins for a delightful and wholesome treat!

Lemon Blueberry Almond Flour Muffins:

Ingredients:

- 2 cups almond flour
- 1/4 cup coconut flour
- 1/4 cup arrowroot flour
- 1 teaspoon baking soda
- 1/4 teaspoon salt
- Zest of 1 lemon
- 3 large eggs
- 1/4 cup honey or agave nectar
- 1/3 cup unsweetened applesauce
- 1/4 cup almond milk
- 1 teaspoon vanilla extract
- 1 cup fresh blueberries

Preparation:

Preheat the oven to 350°F (175°C) and line a muffin tin with paper liners or grease each cup with coconut oil.

In a large bowl, combine almond flour, coconut flour, arrowroot flour, baking soda, salt, and lemon zest.

In a separate bowl, whisk together eggs, honey (or agave nectar), unsweetened applesauce, almond milk, and vanilla extract.

Gradually add the wet ingredients to the dry ingredients, stirring until well combined.

Gently fold in the fresh blueberries.

Fill each muffin cup with the batter, about 3/4 full.

Bake the muffins in the preheated oven for 20-25 minutes or until a toothpick inserted into the center comes out clean.

Allow the muffins to cool in the pan for a few minutes before transferring them to a wire rack to cool completely. Relish the delightful combination of lemon and blueberry in these almond flour muffins!

Cinnamon Swirl Blueberry Almond Flour Muffins:

Ingredients:

- 2 cups almond flour
- 1/4 cup coconut flour
- 1 teaspoon baking powder
- 1/4 teaspoon baking soda
- 1/4 teaspoon salt
- 1 teaspoon ground cinnamon
- 3 large eggs
- 1/4 cup honey or maple syrup
- 1/4 cup unsweetened applesauce
- 1/4 cup almond milk
- 1 teaspoon vanilla extract
- 1 cup fresh blueberries

Preparation:

Preheat the oven to 350°F (175°C) and line a muffin tin with paper liners or grease each cup with coconut oil.

In a mixing bowl, whisk together almond flour, coconut flour, baking powder, baking soda, salt, and ground cinnamon.

In another bowl, whisk the eggs, honey (or maple syrup), unsweetened applesauce, almond milk, and vanilla extract until smooth.

Gradually add the wet ingredients to the dry ingredients, stirring until a smooth batter forms.

Gently fold in the fresh blueberries, distributing them evenly throughout the batter.

Fill each muffin cup with the batter, about 3/4 full.

For the cinnamon swirl, mix together 1 tablespoon of ground cinnamon and 2 tablespoons of honey or maple syrup in a small bowl.

Add a small dollop of the cinnamon swirl mixture on top of each muffin batter and use a toothpick to swirl it in for a marbled effect.

Bake the muffins in the preheated oven for 20-25 minutes or until a toothpick inserted into the center comes out clean.

Allow the muffins to cool in the pan for a few minutes before transferring them to a wire rack to cool completely. Savor the delightful blend of cinnamon and blueberry in these almond flour muffins!

Orange Glazed Blueberry Almond Flour Muffins:

Ingredients:

- 2 cups almond flour
- 1/4 cup coconut flour

- 1/4 cup tapioca flour
- 1 teaspoon baking soda
- 1/4 teaspoon salt
- Zest of 1 orange
- 3 large eggs
- 1/4 cup honey or agave nectar
- 1/4 cup coconut oil, melted
- 1/4 cup freshly squeezed orange juice
- 1 teaspoon vanilla extract
- 1 cup fresh blueberries

Preparation:

Preheat the oven to 350°F (175°C) and line a muffin tin with paper liners or grease each cup with coconut oil.

In a large bowl, mix together almond flour, coconut flour, tapioca flour, baking soda, salt, and orange zest.

In a separate bowl, whisk eggs, honey (or agave nectar), melted coconut oil, orange juice, and vanilla extract.

Gradually add the wet ingredients to the dry ingredients, stirring until well combined.

Gently fold in the fresh blueberries, ensuring an even distribution throughout the batter.

Fill each muffin cup with the batter, about 3/4 full.

Bake the muffins in the preheated oven for 20-25 minutes or until a toothpick inserted into the center comes out clean.

While the muffins are baking, prepare the orange glaze by mixing together 1/4 cup of powdered sugar and 1 tablespoon of freshly squeezed orange juice in a small bowl.

Once the muffins are done, allow them to cool in the pan for a few minutes before transferring them to a wire rack to cool completely. Drizzle the orange glaze over the muffins for a burst of citrusy sweetness!

Double Chocolate Blueberry Almond Flour Muffins:

Ingredients:

- 2 cups almond flour
- 1/4 cup cocoa powder
- 1 teaspoon baking soda
- 1/4 teaspoon salt
- 3 large eggs
- 1/4 cup honey or maple syrup
- 1/4 cup coconut oil, melted
- 1/4 cup almond milk
- 1 teaspoon vanilla extract
- 1/2 cup dark chocolate chips
- 1 cup fresh blueberries

Preparation:

Preheat the oven to 350°F (175°C) and line a muffin tin with paper liners or grease each cup with coconut oil.

In a large mixing bowl, whisk together almond flour, cocoa powder, baking soda, and salt until well combined.

In a separate bowl, whisk the eggs, honey (or maple syrup), melted coconut oil, almond milk, and vanilla extract until smooth.

Gradually add the wet ingredients to the dry ingredients, stirring until a smooth batter forms.

Gently fold in the dark chocolate chips and fresh blueberries, distributing them evenly throughout the batter.

Fill each muffin cup with the batter, about 3/4 full.

Bake the muffins in the preheated oven for 20-25 minutes or until a toothpick inserted into the center comes out clean.

Allow the muffins to cool in the pan for a few minutes before transferring them to a wire rack to cool completely. Delight in the rich chocolaty goodness combined with bursts of juicy blueberries in these almond flour muffins!

Enjoy these scrumptious Almond Flour Blueberry Muffins recipes that not only taste indulgent but also provide a healthier alternative to traditional muffins. With the delightful sweetness of blueberries and the wholesome goodness of almond flour, these muffins are a perfect treat to start your day or enjoy as a delightful snack any time!

Chapter 7

Hydrating Beverages and Refreshing Drinks

Staying well-hydrated is essential for maintaining overall health and vitality, and there's no better way to do it than by indulging in a variety of hydrating beverages and refreshing drinks. Whether you're looking to cool down on a scorching day or add a burst of flavor to your daily hydration routine, these beverages are sure to satisfy your thirst while keeping you feeling energized and revitalized.

Infused Waters: Jazz Up Your H2O

Infused waters are a fantastic way to elevate your hydration game with minimal effort. Simply add slices of your favorite fruits, such as lemon, cucumber, strawberries, or mint leaves, to a pitcher of cold water and let it infuse for a few hours. The result is a naturally flavored and refreshing drink that not only keeps you hydrated but also packs a delightful taste. Experiment with various fruit combinations to find your perfect blend!

Iced Herbal Teas: A Soothing Sip

Herbal teas, served over ice, are a fantastic way to enjoy the benefits of herbs while staying hydrated. Opt for caffeine-free options like chamomile, peppermint, or hibiscus, which not only taste delightful but also offer various health benefits. Brew a large batch, chill it in the fridge, and enjoy a soothing, ice-cold herbal tea whenever you need a moment of relaxation.

Fresh Fruit Smoothies: A Nutrient-Packed Treat

Whip up a refreshing smoothie using a variety of fresh fruits and veggies. Blend together your favorite fruits like bananas, berries, mangoes, and leafy greens with almond milk or coconut water for a hydrating and nutrient-packed beverage. Add a splash of lime or lemon juice for a zesty twist. Smoothies are not only a delicious way to hydrate but also a great option for getting your daily dose of vitamins and minerals.

Sparkling Water Infusions: Effervescent and Flavorful

If you enjoy the fizziness of carbonated beverages, opt for sparkling water infused with natural flavors. Add slices of citrus fruits, crushed berries, or a sprig of fresh herbs to sparkling water for a delightful and hydrating alternative to sugary sodas. The effervescence of sparkling water can make hydration feel like a treat, without any added sugars or artificial ingredients.

Electrolyte Drinks: Replenish and Revitalize

Electrolyte drinks are perfect for rehydrating after exercise or during hot weather when your body loses essential minerals through sweat. You can make your own electrolyte drink by combining water, a pinch of sea salt, a splash of orange juice, and a teaspoon of honey. This simple concoction helps to restore electrolyte balance, keeping you energized and hydrated throughout the day.

Remember, staying hydrated doesn't have to be monotonous. With these hydrating beverages and refreshing drinks, you can elevate your hydration routine and keep yourself feeling revitalized, nourished, and ready to take on whatever the day brings. So, raise a glass to good health and enjoy the delightful flavors of these thirst-quenching concoctions! Cheers to a well-hydrated and vibrant you!

Citrus Infused Water

If you're looking for a delightful and refreshing way to stay hydrated, look no further than citrus-infused water. With just a few simple ingredients, you can transform plain water into a tantalizing, flavor-packed beverage that not only quenches your thirst but also offers a host of health benefits.

Citrus fruits such as lemons, limes, oranges, and grapefruits are bursting with natural flavors and essential nutrients. When infused in water, they release their zesty and aromatic essence, creating a refreshing and invigorating drink that makes hydration a treat for your taste buds.

To make citrus-infused water, simply follow these easy steps:

Choose Your Citrus: Select your favorite citrus fruits or a combination of different ones. Lemons and limes add a tangy and refreshing twist, while oranges bring a hint of sweetness. Grapefruits offer a unique blend of tartness and sweetness, making them a fantastic addition as well.

Slice and Squeeze: Wash the citrus fruits thoroughly and slice them into thin rounds or wedges. Gently squeeze the slices to release some of their juices, which will enhance the flavor of the water.

Infuse the Water: Fill a pitcher or a large glass jar with cold water. Add the citrus slices and any squeezed juice to the water. For a more intense flavor, muddle the citrus slices slightly with a wooden spoon.

Chill and Let Infuse: Refrigerate the water for at least an hour to allow the flavors to infuse fully. For a stronger taste, you can leave the water in the fridge overnight.

The result is a revitalizing and low-calorie beverage that not only helps you stay hydrated but also provides a myriad of health benefits. Citrus fruits are rich in vitamin C, which supports a healthy immune system, aids in collagen production for glowing skin, and helps with the absorption of iron from plant-based sources. Additionally, the natural antioxidants present in citrus fruits help combat free radicals, promoting overall well-being.

Citrus-infused water is a great alternative to sugary sodas and fruit juices, making it an excellent choice for those looking to cut down on their sugar intake. Plus, it's an ideal companion for hot summer days or post-workout rehydration, as the tangy flavors provide a refreshing and revitalizing sensation.

So, the next time you reach for a drink, consider opting for citrus-infused water. Not only will it quench your thirst, but it will also provide a burst of flavor and a healthy dose of nutrients. Experiment with different citrus combinations to find your perfect infusion and raise a glass to the simple pleasure of citrus-infused hydration! Cheers to a refreshing and healthy way to stay hydrated!

Green Tea with Lemon and Ginger

Green tea with lemon and ginger is a delightful and invigorating beverage that combines the goodness of green tea with the tangy zest of lemon and the warm spice of ginger. This harmonious blend not only tantalizes your taste buds but also offers a plethora of health benefits, making it a perfect addition to your daily routine.

Green tea is renowned for its rich antioxidants, particularly catechins like epigallocatechin gallate (EGCG), which have been associated with various health benefits. EGCG is known for its potential to support weight management, boost metabolism, and promote cardiovascular health. It also possesses anti-inflammatory properties, which may aid in reducing the risk of chronic diseases.

Lemon adds a burst of Vitamin C to the mix, enhancing the tea's antioxidant power while imparting a refreshing and tangy flavor. Vitamin C is a potent antioxidant that supports the immune system, aids in collagen production for healthy skin, and helps the body absorb iron from plant-based sources.

Ginger, on the other hand, brings its own array of benefits to the table. This warming spice is revered for its anti-inflammatory and digestive properties. It can help soothe upset stomachs, alleviate nausea, and promote overall gut health.

To prepare green tea with lemon and ginger:

1. Boil water and let it cool for a few minutes (green tea should be brewed at around 175°F or 80°C for the best flavor).

2. Add a green tea bag or loose green tea leaves to a teapot or cup.
3. Slice a few thin rounds of fresh lemon and a small piece of fresh ginger.
4. Add the lemon slices and ginger to the teapot or cup.
5. Pour the hot water over the tea bag or leaves, lemon, and ginger.
6. Allow the tea to steep for 2-3 minutes for a milder flavor or up to 5 minutes for a stronger brew.
7. Remove the tea bag or strain the loose tea leaves, lemon, and ginger from the tea.
8. Optionally, you can add a touch of honey or maple syrup for a hint of sweetness.

The result is a rejuvenating and aromatic cup of green tea with lemon and ginger, packed with antioxidants and delightful flavors. It's a perfect pick-me-up in the morning or a soothing treat to unwind after a long day.

Apart from its various health benefits, this beverage is also a calorie-conscious choice, making it an excellent alternative to sugary beverages. By incorporating green tea with lemon and ginger into your daily routine, you not only get to enjoy a delightful and refreshing drink but also reap the rewards of its nourishing properties.

So, next time you're looking for a revitalizing and healthful beverage, consider brewing a cup of green tea with lemon and ginger. Sip and savor the harmonious blend of flavors, knowing that you're indulging in a drink that not only tastes fantastic but also supports your overall well-being. Cheers to the goodness of green tea, lemon, and ginger!

Cucumber Mint Cooler

The cucumber mint cooler is a delightful and cooling beverage that is perfect for quenching your thirst on hot summer days. This refreshing concoction combines the hydrating properties of cucumber with the invigorating essence of mint, creating a drink that not only refreshes your body but also rejuvenates your senses.

Cucumbers are composed mainly of water, making them an excellent choice for staying hydrated. They are low in calories and rich in vitamins and minerals, including vitamin K, vitamin C, potassium, and magnesium. Cucumbers also contain antioxidants, such as beta-carotene and flavonoids, which contribute to their health benefits.

Mint, on the other hand, is known for its invigorating aroma and distinct flavor. It adds a refreshing twist to the cucumber cooler while offering its own set of health benefits. Mint has been traditionally used to aid digestion, relieve indigestion and bloating, and soothe an upset stomach. Additionally, it contains menthol, which provides a cooling sensation and can help alleviate headaches and ease respiratory discomfort.

To prepare the cucumber mint cooler:

1. Wash and peel a fresh cucumber, then cut it into slices.
2. In a blender, combine the cucumber slices with a handful of fresh mint leaves.
3. Add a splash of fresh lime or lemon juice for a tangy kick.
4. Optionally, you can add a teaspoon of honey or agave syrup for a touch of sweetness.
5. Blend the ingredients until smooth.
6. Pour the mixture into a glass filled with ice cubes.
7. Garnish with a sprig of fresh mint or a cucumber slice, and enjoy your cool and revitalizing cucumber mint cooler!

This delightful beverage is not only refreshing but also incredibly versatile. You can experiment with different variations by adding ingredients like ginger, basil, or even a hint of sparkling water for a fizzy twist. It's a fantastic non-alcoholic option for picnics, barbecues, or any summer gathering.

Moreover, the cucumber mint cooler is a healthy and hydrating alternative to sugary sodas and artificial drinks. It's a low-calorie option that supports your hydration needs and provides a burst of natural flavors and nutrients.

So, the next time you want to beat the heat and treat yourself to a revitalizing drink, whip up a batch of cucumber mint cooler. Embrace the cool and refreshing sensation as you sip this rejuvenating elixir. Cheers to a summer sip that not only cools you down but also nourishes your body and soul!

Chapter 8

Meal Planning and Grocery Shopping Tips

Meal planning and grocery shopping might seem like mundane tasks, but they play a crucial role in nourishing your body and maintaining a healthy lifestyle. By adopting smart strategies and efficient approaches, you can transform these routines into enjoyable and rewarding experiences. Here are some valuable tips to help you streamline your meal planning and grocery shopping, ensuring you make nutritious choices without feeling overwhelmed.

1. Plan Ahead for Success: Start by dedicating some time each week to plan your meals. Create a weekly or bi-weekly meal plan that includes breakfast, lunch, dinner, and snacks. Consider your dietary preferences, nutritional needs, and any specific health goals. Planning ahead not only saves time but also reduces food waste and helps you make healthier choices.

2. Embrace Variety: Maintaining a balanced diet requires a diverse range of foods. Incorporate fruits, vegetables, whole grains, lean proteins, and healthy fats into your meal plan. Experiment with new recipes and ingredients to keep your meals exciting and enjoyable.

3. Make a Detailed Grocery List: Based on your meal plan, create a comprehensive grocery

list. Organize it by categories, such as produce, dairy, pantry staples, and frozen foods. Having a well-organized list will streamline your shopping and prevent you from forgetting essential items.

4. Shop the Perimeter: When navigating the grocery store, focus on the perimeter where fresh produce, lean meats, dairy, and whole grains are typically located. Minimize your time in the processed food aisles, which are often filled with sugary and unhealthy choices.

5. Read Labels Mindfully: While shopping, take the time to read food labels carefully. Look for items with minimal added sugars, sodium, and unhealthy fats. Opt for whole, unprocessed foods whenever possible.

6. Buy in Bulk: Stock up on non-perishable items, like whole grains, legumes, and nuts, by buying in bulk. Not only does this save money, but it also ensures you always have nutritious ingredients on hand.

7. Choose Seasonal Produce: Seasonal fruits and vegetables are often fresher, more flavorful, and less expensive. Build your meal plan around what's in season to support local agriculture and enjoy the best quality produce.

8. Shop with a Full Stomach: Avoid grocery shopping on an empty stomach to resist the temptation of impulse buys. When you shop

while hungry, you may be more likely to grab unhealthy snacks and treats.

9. Utilize Online Shopping: Take advantage of online grocery shopping and delivery services, which can save you time and reduce impulse purchases. Many stores offer these services, making it easier than ever to shop efficiently.

10. Be Mindful of Portion Sizes: When purchasing items like grains, nuts, and dried fruits, be mindful of portion sizes to prevent overconsumption. Pre-portioning these items at home can help control your intake and reduce waste.

By implementing these meal planning and grocery shopping tips, you can ensure that you nourish your body with nutritious foods while making the process efficient and enjoyable. Empower yourself to create wholesome meals that support your well-being and align with your health goals. Happy meal planning and shopping!

Creating a Weekly Meal Plan

Meal planning is a powerful tool that can transform your eating habits and streamline your daily routine. By dedicating a little time each week to plan your meals, you set yourself up for success, nourishing your body with balanced and nutritious foods while saving time, money, and stress. Here's a step-by-step guide to help you create a weekly meal plan that fits your lifestyle and dietary preferences.

1. Assess Your Needs: Begin by evaluating your dietary needs and goals. Consider any dietary restrictions, preferences, or health objectives you want to achieve. Whether you're following a specific diet, aiming to lose weight, or simply looking to eat more wholesome foods, identifying your goals will guide your meal planning decisions.

2. Plan Your Meals: Using a weekly calendar or a meal planning app, outline your meals for each day of the week. Start with breakfast, lunch, dinner, and snacks. Aim for a variety of foods, incorporating fruits, vegetables, whole grains, lean proteins, and healthy fats into each meal.

3. Think About Convenience: Take into account your schedule and lifestyle when planning meals. On busy days, opt for quick and easy recipes that require minimal preparation. Consider leftovers or meal prepping to save time on hectic days.

4. Make a Grocery List: Based on your meal plan, create a detailed grocery list. Organize it by categories like produce, dairy, proteins, pantry staples, and snacks. This will make your shopping experience more efficient and prevent you from forgetting essential items.

5. Shop with Intention: Head to the grocery store with your list in hand and stick to it. Avoid impulsive purchases of unhealthy snacks or treats that may derail your meal plan.

6. Be Flexible: While a meal plan provides structure, don't be afraid to be flexible. Life happens, and plans may change. Allow yourself room to swap meals or ingredients if needed.

7. Use Seasonal Produce: Incorporate seasonal fruits and vegetables into your meal plan. Not only are they fresher and more flavorful, but they're also often more affordable.

8. Avoid Food Waste: Consider using ingredients that can be used in multiple meals throughout the week. This reduces food waste and saves money.

9. Batch Cook and Freeze: If your schedule allows, batch cook certain recipes and freeze portions for later in the week. This way, you can enjoy homemade meals without spending hours in the kitchen each day.

10. Embrace Variety: Don't be afraid to try new recipes and experiment with different flavors

and cuisines. Embracing variety in your meal plan keeps things exciting and enjoyable.

Creating a weekly meal plan is a game-changer for your health and well-being. It empowers you to take control of your nutrition, make mindful food choices, and reduce stress around mealtime. With a well-planned menu, you can savor delicious, nourishing meals while supporting your overall health and fitness goals. So, grab a pen and paper, and start crafting your personalized recipe for success with a weekly meal plan!

Stocking Your Pantry with Low-GI Essentials

Stocking your pantry with low-GI essentials is a smart and proactive way to support your health and maintain stable blood sugar levels. The glycemic index (GI) ranks carbohydrates based on how they affect blood glucose levels. Low-GI foods have a slow and gradual impact on blood sugar, making them ideal choices for promoting sustained energy and overall well-being. Here's a guide to help you build a pantry filled with nutritious, low-GI essentials.

1. Whole Grains: Whole grains are an excellent foundation for a low-GI pantry. Opt for whole wheat, quinoa, barley, brown rice, and oats. These grains are rich in fiber, vitamins, and minerals, and they provide a steady

release of energy, keeping you satiated and satisfied for longer periods.

2. Legumes and Pulses: Stock up on lentils, chickpeas, black beans, and kidney beans. These legumes are packed with protein, fiber, and essential nutrients, offering a low-GI alternative to refined carbohydrates.

3. Nuts and Seeds: Nuts and seeds are nutrient powerhouses that provide healthy fats, protein, and fiber. Almonds, chia seeds, flaxseeds, and walnuts are great additions to your pantry for adding crunch and nutrition to meals and snacks.

4. Healthy Oils: Choose healthy oils such as olive oil, coconut oil, and avocado oil. These oils provide essential fatty acids and contribute to a well-rounded low-GI pantry.

5. Canned and Dried Fruits: Opt for canned fruits in their natural juice or dried fruits with no added sugars. While fruits have varying GI values, choosing these options ensures you have healthy, natural sweets readily available for your low-GI meal planning.

6. Canned and Dried Vegetables: Keep canned tomatoes, artichokes, and other vegetables on hand for quick and convenient low-GI meal preparation. Dried mushrooms, sun-dried tomatoes, and seaweed are excellent options for adding flavor and variety to your dishes.

7. Low-GI Snacks: Choose snacks that won't spike your blood sugar, such as unsalted nuts,

air-popped popcorn, and roasted chickpeas. These options are tasty and nourishing, making them ideal choices for satisfying cravings between meals.

Nut Butters: Peanut butter, almond butter, and other nut butters are delicious and nutritious additions to your pantry. They're versatile and can be used in smoothies, dressings, and dips, adding creaminess and flavor without compromising your low-GI goals.

Herbs and Spices: Stock up on herbs and spices like cinnamon, turmeric, basil, and oregano. They enhance the taste of your meals while contributing beneficial compounds and antioxidants.

Low-GI Sweeteners: Choose natural sweeteners like stevia, erythritol, and monk fruit for your low-GI pantry. These alternatives provide sweetness without causing rapid spikes in blood sugar levels.

By stocking your pantry with these low-GI essentials, you lay the groundwork for a balanced and nourishing diet. These wholesome ingredients provide sustenance, promote satiety, and support your overall well-being. With a well-prepared pantry, you can effortlessly create delicious low-GI meals that help you maintain steady energy levels and support your health journey. Remember to check labels and choose unprocessed options whenever possible to ensure you're making the best choices for your low-GI pantry.

Tips for Grocery Shopping on a Glycemic Index Diet

Grocery shopping on a Glycemic Index (GI) diet can be a rewarding and health-conscious experience. By selecting low-GI foods, you support stable blood sugar levels and promote overall well-being. Whether you're new to the GI diet or a seasoned pro, these tips will help you navigate the aisles with confidence and make the best choices for your low-GI grocery shopping.

1. Familiarize Yourself with Low-GI Foods: Before heading to the store, familiarize yourself with low-GI foods and their GI values. Focus on whole grains, legumes, non-starchy vegetables, lean proteins, and healthy fats. Opt for fresh, unprocessed options whenever possible to ensure you're selecting the most nutritious choices.

2. Read Food Labels: Take the time to read food labels carefully. Look for foods with a low or moderate GI value (55 or less) and avoid items with high GI values (70 or more). Be mindful of added sugars, as they can increase a food's GI ranking.

3. Shop the Perimeter: When grocery shopping, focus on the perimeter of the store where you'll find fresh produce, lean proteins, and dairy products. The inner aisles often contain processed and high-GI foods, so minimizing your time there can help you stay on track.

4. Opt for Whole Grains: Choose whole grains over refined grains. Look for products labeled "whole grain" or "100% whole wheat." Whole grains have a lower GI value and provide more fiber and nutrients.

5. Stock Up on Vegetables: Load up your cart with a colorful variety of non-starchy vegetables, such as leafy greens, bell peppers, broccoli, and zucchini. These vegetables have a low GI and are rich in vitamins and minerals.

6. Include Lean Proteins: Choose lean proteins like poultry, fish, tofu, and legumes. Protein-rich foods have a minimal effect on blood sugar levels and can help you feel full and satisfied.

7. Limit Processed Foods: Minimize your consumption of processed and packaged foods, as they often have higher GI values and may contain added sugars and unhealthy fats. Opt for whole, unprocessed foods whenever possible.

8. Be Cautious with Fruit: While fruit is generally healthy, some varieties have a higher GI value. Stick to fruits with a lower GI, such as berries, cherries, and apples. Enjoy fruit in moderation and pair it with protein or healthy fats to further balance its impact on blood sugar.

9. Plan Your Meals: Create a meal plan before grocery shopping. Knowing what you need

will help you avoid impulse purchases and stay focused on low-GI options.

10. Shop Mindfully: Avoid shopping when hungry, as it may lead to impulsive and less nutritious choices. Go grocery shopping after eating a meal or snack to stay on track with your low-GI diet.

By following these tips, you can approach grocery shopping on a Glycemic Index diet with confidence and make informed choices that align with your health goals. With a well-stocked cart full of nourishing and low-GI foods, you set yourself up for success on your journey to stable blood sugar levels and improved overall health. Happy low-GI shopping!

Conclusion

As we come to the end of this Glycemic Index Diet Cookbook journey, we celebrate the nourishing and delicious recipes that have graced our tables. The path to balanced living through the Glycemic Index has been an enlightening one, filled with newfound appreciation for the impact of our food choices on our well-being.

Throughout these pages, we've explored the principles of the Glycemic Index, understanding how it influences our blood sugar levels and, ultimately, our health. We've delved into the world of low-GI foods, savoring the abundance of nutrient-rich ingredients that support our bodies from the inside out.

From energizing breakfasts and wholesome lunches to delectable dinners and sweet treats, this cookbook has empowered us to create flavorful meals without sacrificing health or taste. Each recipe has been thoughtfully crafted to include low-GI ingredients, offering a harmonious balance of flavors and nourishment.

But this journey extends beyond the kitchen. It's about embracing a lifestyle that prioritizes mindful eating, self-awareness, and appreciation for the foods that fuel our bodies. It's about recognizing that every meal is an opportunity to nourish and nurture ourselves.

As we move forward, let us carry this newfound knowledge into our daily lives. Let us make conscious choices about the foods we consume, appreciating the power of nutrition in shaping our well-being. Let us remember that small changes in our diets can lead to significant transformations in our health.

The Glycemic Index Diet Cookbook serves as a guide, inspiring us to explore the vast array of low-GI foods and create meals that elevate our health and happiness. Whether you're managing diabetes, seeking sustained energy, or simply embracing a healthier lifestyle, these recipes offer a delicious and fulfilling path.

As we bid farewell, may the recipes shared within these pages continue to grace your tables, bringing joy and nourishment to your life. Remember that the journey toward balanced living is not about perfection, but progress. Embrace the Glycemic Goodness, one mindful bite at a time.

Wishing you vibrant health and a life filled with the goodness of the Glycemic Index.

Appendix A: Glycemic Index Food List

Incorporating the Glycemic Index (GI) into your dietary choices can be a game-changer for your overall health and well-being. By focusing on low-GI foods and making mindful choices, you can support stable blood sugar levels, improve energy levels, and reduce the risk of chronic diseases.

Throughout this journey, you've learned the ins and outs of the Glycemic Index diet, from understanding the concept of GI and its impact on blood sugar to creating balanced meal plans and stocking your pantry with low-GI essentials. Armed with knowledge and practical tips, you can confidently navigate grocery store aisles, choose nutritious foods, and prepare delicious meals that align with your health goals.

In Appendix A, you'll find a comprehensive Glycemic Index Food List, guiding you on the GI values of various foods. This valuable resource will help you make informed decisions when creating your meal plans and grocery shopping lists.

As you continue your low-GI journey, remember that balance and consistency are key. Embrace variety in your diet, experiment with new recipes, and make room for occasional treats while keeping an eye on portion sizes. Stay mindful of the glycemic load, which considers both the GI value and the portion size of a food. Integrating physical activity, stress management, and sufficient sleep into your lifestyle complements your low-GI diet, promoting overall health and vitality.

Your commitment to a low-GI lifestyle can have far-reaching benefits, not only for your physical health but also for your mental and emotional well-being. As you experience the positive impact of balanced blood sugar levels, you'll likely notice increased energy, improved focus, and a greater sense of well-being.

In conclusion, the Glycemic Index diet offers a wealth of benefits, empowering you to take charge of your health and make choices that serve your body and mind. Embrace the principles of the low-GI lifestyle, use the provided resources wisely, and remember that each step toward a healthier you is a step worth celebrating.

Appendix A: Glycemic Index Food List

This appendix contains a comprehensive list of various foods and their corresponding Glycemic Index values. Use it as a reference when planning your meals and grocery shopping to make informed decisions about the foods you choose to nourish your body.

Appendix B: Conversion Tables References Index

In this appendix, you'll find essential conversion tables, a list of references used throughout the book, and a comprehensive index for easy navigation and reference.

Conversion Tables:

1. Measurement Conversions:

- Cups to Milliliters
- Teaspoons to Milliliters
- Tablespoons to Milliliters
- Fahrenheit to Celsius

2. Weight Conversions:

- Pounds to Kilograms
- Ounces to Grams

3. Ingredient Substitutions:

- Common Ingredient Substitutions for Dietary Restrictions

References:

1. Books:

- List of books and scholarly sources referenced in this cookbook.

2. Scientific Journals:

- Credible scientific journals used as references for evidence-based information.

3. Websites:

- Reputable websites and online resources consulted for research and additional information.

Index: The index is a comprehensive guide to finding specific topics, recipes, and relevant information throughout the cookbook. Use it as a quick reference tool to locate what you need quickly and efficiently.

By including these conversion tables, references, and an index, this appendix enhances the functionality and usability of the Glycemic Index Diet Cookbook. It aims to provide you with a seamless and enjoyable experience as you embark on your journey toward a healthier and more balanced lifestyle.

Remember that the information in this book is not a substitute for personalized medical advice. Always consult with a healthcare professional before making significant changes to your diet or lifestyle, especially if you have specific health conditions or concerns.

Happy cooking and bon appétit!

Please note that the recipes and information provided in this book are intended for general informational purposes only and are not a substitute for professional medical advice. Always consult with a qualified healthcare provider or registered dietitian before making significant changes to your diet, especially if you have specific health conditions or dietary needs.

www.ingramcontent.com/pod-product-compliance
Lightning Source LLC
Chambersburg PA
CBHW070946260726
48661CB00003B/1147